1. Salmon with quinoa and steamed broccoli

Ingredients:
- 4 (6 oz) salmon fillets
- 2 tsp olive oil
- Salt and pepper to taste
- 1 cup quinoa, rinsed
- 2 cups low-sodium vegetable or chicken broth
- 1 lb broccoli florets
- 2 tbsp lemon juice
- 2 tbsp chopped fresh parsley

Instructions:

1. Season the salmon fillets with salt, pepper and 1 tsp of the olive oil on both sides.

2. In a saucepan, combine the quinoa and broth. Bring to a boil, then reduce heat to low, cover and simmer for 15-20 minutes until quinoa is tender and liquid is absorbed.

3. Place broccoli in a steamer basket over 1 inch of boiling water in a saucepan. Cover and steam for 5-7 minutes until broccoli is tender-crisp.

4. Heat remaining 1 tsp olive oil in a skillet over medium-high heat. Add salmon fillets and cook for 4-5 minutes per side until cooked through and lightly browned on both sides.

5. Fluff quinoa with a fork and stir in lemon juice and parsley. Season with salt and pepper to taste.

6. Serve salmon fillets over quinoa with the steamed broccoli on the side. Drizzle any extra lemon juice over the salmon and broccoli if desired.

This healthy meal provides protein from the salmon, fiber and nutrients from the quinoa and broccoli. The lemon and parsley add freshness. Adjust cooking times as needed for desired doneness.

2. Turmeric-spiced lentil soup

Ingredients:
- 1 tbsp olive oil
- 1 onion, diced
- 3 cloves garlic, minced
- 1 tbsp grated fresh ginger
- 1 tsp ground turmeric
- 1 tsp ground cumin
- 1⁄4 tsp cayenne pepper (or to taste)
- 4 cups vegetable or chicken broth
- 1 cup dried green or brown lentils, rinsed
- 1 (14.5 oz) can diced tomatoes
- 2 cups chopped kale or spinach
- 2 tbsp lemon juice
- Salt and pepper to taste
- Chopped cilantro for garnish

Instructions:

1. In a large pot, heat the olive oil over medium heat. Add the onions and sauté for 5 minutes until translucent.

2. Add the garlic, ginger, turmeric, cumin and cayenne. Cook for 1 minute until fragrant.

3. Pour in the broth and lentils. Bring to a boil, then reduce heat and simmer for 15-20 minutes, until lentils are tender.

4. Add the diced tomatoes with juices and the chopped greens. Simmer 5 more minutes.

5. Remove soup from heat and stir in the lemon juice. Season to taste with salt and pepper.

6. Ladle soup into bowls and garnish with chopped cilantro.

For a creamier soup, use an immersion blender to partially puree a portion of the soup. You can also add a dollop of plain yogurt when serving.

This flavorful, protein-packed vegan soup features the warm spices of turmeric and cumin along with the bright notes of ginger and lemon. It's hearty, nutritious and easy to make.

Welcome to ***"The Psoriatic Arthritis Diet Cookbook: 100+ Recipes for Happy Joints"***. This book is your essential companion on the journey to managing psoriatic arthritis through the power of nutrition. Whether you've recently been diagnosed or have been living with psoriatic arthritis for years, adopting a healthy diet tailored to your condition can significantly improve your quality of life.

Psoriatic arthritis is a chronic autoimmune condition that affects the joints and often accompanies psoriasis, a skin condition characterized by red, scaly patches. Managing psoriatic arthritis requires a comprehensive approach that includes medication, lifestyle changes, and dietary modifications. While there is no one-size-fits-all diet for psoriatic arthritis, certain foods have been shown to help reduce inflammation, alleviate symptoms, and support joint health.

This cookbook is designed to provide you with a diverse array of delicious recipes that are not only satisfying to the palate but also gentle on your joints. Each recipe has been carefully crafted to incorporate ingredients known for their anti-inflammatory properties, helping you nourish your body and support your joint health.

In addition to the recipes, this book offers valuable insights into the role of diet in managing psoriatic arthritis. You'll learn about specific foods that can help reduce inflammation, tips for meal planning and preparation, and practical strategies for incorporating these foods into your daily routine. Whether you're a seasoned home cook or new to the kitchen, you'll find inspiration and guidance to help you create nourishing meals that support your health and well-being.

Here's what you can expect from this book:

- ***100+ Delicious Recipes:*** Explore a variety of recipes for every meal and occasion, from vibrant salads and hearty soups to flavorful main courses and decadent desserts. Each recipe is designed to be both nutritious and delicious, making it easy to enjoy healthy eating.

- ***Anti-Inflammatory Ingredients:*** Discover the power of ingredients that can help reduce inflammation and support joint health, such as omega-3 fatty acids, antioxidants, and anti-inflammatory spices and herbs.

- ***Practical Tips and Advice:*** Learn practical strategies for shopping, meal planning, and cooking to make healthy eating a seamless part of your lifestyle. Whether you're cooking for yourself or for the whole family, you'll find tips to help you save time and effort in the kitchen.

- Scientific Insights: Gain a better understanding of the connection between diet and psoriatic arthritis with clear explanations of the latest research. Empower yourself with knowledge to make informed decisions about your diet and lifestyle.

This cookbook is more than just a collection of recipes; it's a comprehensive resource for anyone looking to take control of their health and well-being with delicious, arthritis-friendly meals. We hope that the recipes and insights provided in this book will inspire you to nourish your body, soothe inflammation, and enjoy a life of happy joints.

Thank you for choosing ***"The Psoriatic Arthritis Diet Cookbook: 100+ Recipes for Happy Joints"*** as your guide to healthier living. Let's embark on this culinary journey together and discover the joy of eating well for better health.

Warm regards,

Gustav Henning

Author of "The Psoriatic Arthritis Diet Cookbook: 100+ Recipes for Happy Joints"

3. Grilled chicken salad with mixed greens and avocado

Ingredients:
- 4 (6oz) boneless, skinless chicken breasts
- 2 tbsp olive oil, plus more for brushing
- Juice of 1 lemon
- 1 tsp dried oregano
- Salt and pepper to taste
- 8 cups mixed greens (romaine, arugula, spinach)
- 1 avocado, pitted and sliced
- 1 cucumber, diced
- 1 cup cherry tomatoes, halved
- 1/4 cup sliced red onion
- 1/4 cup fresh parsley, chopped

Dressing:
- 1/4 cup olive oil
- 2 tbsp red wine vinegar
- 1 tbsp Dijon mustard
- 1 garlic clove, minced
- Salt and pepper to taste

Instructions:
1. In a shallow dish, combine 2 tbsp olive oil, lemon juice, oregano, salt and pepper. Add chicken and turn to coat. Let marinate for 30 minutes.

2. Preheat grill or grill pan to medium-high heat. Brush grill grates with oil. Grill chicken 5-7 minutes per side until cooked through. Let rest 5 minutes then slice.

3. Make the dressing by whisking together olive oil, vinegar, mustard, garlic, salt and pepper.

4. In a large bowl, toss the mixed greens with the cucumber, tomatoes, onion, parsley and half the dressing.

5. Divide salad among 4 plates and top each with sliced avocado and grilled chicken slices. Drizzle remaining dressing over the top.

This salad contains ingredients that may help reduce inflammation associated with psoriatic arthritis like healthy fats from olive oil and avocado, antioxidants from the vegetables and herbs, and lean protein from the grilled chicken. The mixed greens provide fiber, vitamins and minerals as well. Adjust ingredients as needed for dietary needs.

4. Vegetable stir-fry with tofu

Ingredients:
- 14 oz extra-firm tofu, drained and cubed
- 2 tbsp soy sauce or tamari, divided
- 2 tbsp rice vinegar
- 1 tbsp sesame oil
- 1 tbsp cornstarch
- 2 tbsp vegetable or canola oil
- 1 red bell pepper, sliced
- 1 cup broccoli florets
- 1 cup sliced mushrooms
- 1 cup snap or snow peas
- 3 cloves garlic, minced
- 1 tbsp grated fresh ginger
- 4 green onions, sliced, whites and greens separated
- Cooked brown rice or quinoa, for serving

Instructions:

1. Place the cubed tofu in a shallow bowl and toss with 1 tbsp soy sauce or tamari. Let marinate for 10-15 minutes.

2. In a small bowl, whisk together the vinegar, remaining 1 tbsp soy sauce, sesame oil, and cornstarch. Set aside.

3. Heat vegetable oil in a large skillet or wok over high heat. Add the marinated tofu and stir-fry for 2 minutes until lightly browned on all sides. Transfer tofu to a plate.

4. Add the bell pepper, broccoli, mushrooms, and snap peas to the skillet. Stir-fry for 3 minutes.

5. Add the garlic, ginger, and white parts of the green onions. Stir-fry for 1 minute more.

6. Whisk the soy sauce mixture again to re-incorporate the cornstarch, then pour into the skillet. Toss to coat the vegetables.

7. Return the tofu to the skillet and stir everything together. Cook for 1-2 minutes until the sauce thickens up slightly.

8. Remove from heat and stir in the green parts of the onions. Serve immediately over steamed brown rice or quinoa.

This meatless stir-fry is packed with protein from the tofu and lots of fresh, crisp-tender veggies. The light sauce gives it classic Asian flavor. Feel free to sub in other vegetables you have on hand like carrots, cabbage, bean sprouts or water chestnuts. A quick and healthy plant-based meal!

5. Spinach and mushroom omelette

Ingredients:
- 3 eggs
- 1 tbsp water or milk
- 1/4 tsp salt
- 1/8 tsp black pepper
- 1 tsp butter or olive oil
- 1/2 cup sliced mushrooms (button, cremini, etc.)
- 1 clove garlic, minced
- 2 cups fresh baby spinach
- 2 tbsp crumbled feta or goat cheese (optional)

Instructions:
1. Crack the eggs into a small bowl and add the water/milk, salt and pepper. Beat lightly with a fork until blended.

2. Heat a small non-stick skillet over medium heat and add the butter/oil. Once melted, add the sliced mushrooms and sauté for 2-3 minutes until starting to brown.

3. Add the minced garlic and sauté for 30 seconds until fragrant.

4. Add the fresh spinach leaves and continue cooking for 1-2 minutes, turning occasionally, until the spinach is wilted down.

5. Pour in the beaten eggs and tilt the pan to spread them evenly over the mushroom spinach mixture.

6. As the eggs begin to set, use a spatula to gently push the cooked edges towards the center, allowing the uncooked eggs to flow to the outer edges.

7. Once the bottom is set but the top is still a bit runny, sprinkle the cheese (if using) over half of the omelette.

8. Fold the other half over and slide the omelette onto a plate. Let sit for 1 minute before serving hot.

This veggie-packed omelette makes a satisfying, protein-rich breakfast. The mushrooms add an earthy flavor while the spinach provides nutrients. The feta or goat cheese adds a creamy, tangy note. For extra flavor, serve with sliced avocado, salsa or hot sauce on the side.

6. Baked sweet potato with black beans and salsa

Ingredients:
- 4 medium sweet potatoes, scrubbed clean
- 1 (15 oz) can black beans, drained and rinsed
- 1 tsp ground cumin
- 1/4 tsp chili powder
- 1 cup salsa, plus more for serving
- 1/2 cup shredded cheddar or pepper jack cheese
- 2 green onions, thinly sliced
- Fresh cilantro for garnish
- Plain Greek yogurt or sour cream (optional)

Instructions:

1. Preheat oven to 400°F. Prick the sweet potatoes several times with a fork and place on a foil-lined baking sheet.

2. Bake for 50-60 minutes, until easily pierced with a fork. Allow to cool slightly.

3. In a small saucepan, combine the drained black beans, cumin and chili powder. Heat through over medium, mashing some of the beans to thicken it slightly if desired.

4. Once cool enough to handle, slice each sweet potato lengthwise and fluff the insides with a fork.

5. Top each potato half with a spoonful of the warm black bean mixture, then salsa, shredded cheese and sliced green onions.

6. Return to the oven for 5 minutes until cheese is melted.

7. Remove and garnish with cilantro. Serve immediately with extra salsa and Greek yogurt/sour cream if desired.

The sweet potato base provides nutrients, fiber and healthy carbs while the black bean and salsa topping adds protein, vegetables, spice and Mexican-inspired flavors. This satisfying vegetarian meal is easy to prepare and highly customizable with your favorite salsa and toppings. Leftovers als reheat well for quick meals later.

7. Lentil and vegetable curry

Ingredients:
- 1 cup dried green or brown lentils, rinsed
- 1 tbsp olive oil
- 1 onion, diced
- 3 cloves garlic, minced
- 1 tbsp grated fresh ginger
- 1-2 tsp curry powder
- 1 tsp ground cumin
- 1 tsp ground coriander
- 1⁄4 tsp cayenne pepper (or to taste)
- 1 (14 oz) can diced tomatoes
- 4 cups vegetable or chicken broth
- 2 cups cauliflower florets
- 2 carrots, sliced
- 1 cup frozen peas
- Salt and pepper to taste
- Chopped cilantro for garnish

Instructions:

1. In a large pot, cover the lentils with water and bring to a boil. Reduce heat and simmer for 5 minutes. Drain and set aside.

2. In the same pot, heat the olive oil over medium heat. Add the onions and sauté for 5 minutes until translucent.

3. Add the garlic, ginger, curry powder, cumin, coriander and cayenne. Cook for 1 minute until fragrant.

4. Stir in the diced tomatoes with juices, broth, lentils, cauliflower and carrots. Bring to a boil.

5. Reduce heat to low, cover and simmer for 15-20 minutes until lentils and vegetables are tender.

6. Stir in the frozen peas and season to taste with salt and pepper.

7. Ladle the curry into bowls and garnish with chopped cilantro.

For added richness, stir in a dollop of plain yogurt when serving. Serve over basmati rice or with naan bread on the side.

This hearty, flavorful curry makes a satisfying vegetarian meal loaded with plant-based protein from the lentils and veggies. It's easy to make and great for meal prep.

8. Quinoa stuffed bell peppers

Ingredients:

- 1 cup corn kernels (frozen or fresh)
- 1 (15 oz) can black beans,
drained and rinsed
- 1 tsp cumin
- 1 tsp chili powder
- 1/2 cup shredded cheddar or
Mexican blend cheese
- 2 tbsp chopped fresh cilantro
- Salt and pepper to taste

- 4 large bell peppers (any color),
tops cut off and seeded
- 1 cup quinoa, rinsed
- 2 cups vegetable or chicken broth
- 1 tbsp olive oil
- 1/2 onion, diced
- 2 cloves garlic, minced
- 1 cup diced mushrooms

Instructions:

1. Preheat oven to 375°F. Cut tops off peppers and remove seeds and membranes. Place peppers in a baking dish and set aside.

2. In a saucepan, combine quinoa and broth. Bring to a boil, then reduce heat to low. Simmer covered for 15-20 minutes until liquid is absorbed. Fluff with a fork.

3. In a skillet, heat the olive oil over medium-high heat. Sauté the onion for 2-3 minutes until translucent.

4. Add the garlic and mushrooms and cook 2 more minutes.

5. Stir in the cooked quinoa, black beans, corn, cumin, chili powder and salt and pepper to taste.

6. Remove from heat and stir in the cheese and cilantro, reserving some for topping.

7. Fill each hollowed pepper cavity with the quinoa mixture.

8. Cover baking dish with foil and bake for 30 minutes.

9. Uncover, top with remaining cheese and bake 10 more minutes until heated through.

10. Garnish with remaining cilantro before serving.

These protein-packed stuffed peppers are vegetarian, nutritious and full of southwestern flavors. They make a great meat-free main dish or can be served as a tasty side. Feel free to swap in other veggies you have on hand. Leftover filling also makes a great burrito or salad topping.

9. Grilled shrimp skewers with roasted vegetables

Ingredients:
- 1 lb large shrimp, peeled and deveined
- 2 tbsp olive oil, plus more for vegetables
- 2 cloves garlic, minced
- 1 tsp paprika
- 1/2 tsp dried oregano
- Zest of 1 lemon
- Salt and pepper to taste
- 1 zucchini, cut into 1-inch chunks
- 1 red bell pepper, cut into 1-inch pieces
- 1/2 red onion, cut into wedges
- 8-10 cherry tomatoes
- 2 tbsp lemon juice
- Chopped parsley for garnish

Instructions:
1. Soak 8-10 wooden skewers in water for 30 minutes to prevent burning.

2. In a bowl, toss the shrimp with 2 tbsp olive oil, garlic, paprika, oregano, lemon zest and salt and pepper. Cover and marinate for 15-30 minutes.

3. Preheat oven to 400°F. On a baking sheet, toss the zucchini, bell pepper, onion and tomatoes with olive oil and season with salt and pepper.

4. Roast vegetables for 15-20 minutes, tossing halfway, until tender and lightly charred.

5. Meanwhile, thread the shrimp onto the soaked skewers, leaving a bit of space between each one.

6. Preheat grill or grill pan to medium-high heat and brush grates with oil.

7. Grill shrimp skewers for 2-3 minutes per side until charred and opaque throughout.

8. Transfer roasted vegetables to a platter and squeeze fresh lemon juice over top. Arrange grilled shrimp skewers over vegetables. Garnish with chopped parsley and serve immediately with extra lemon wedges if desired.

These grilled shrimp skewers and oven-roasted vegetables make a light, healthy and flavorful summertime meal. The lemon, garlic and oregano give the shrimp plenty of bright flavor. You can mix up the veggie combination based on your preference. Serve with crusty bread or over pasta or rice if desired.

10. Chickpea salad with cucumber and tomato

Ingredients:
- 1 (15oz) can chickpeas, drained and rinsed
- 1 cucumber, diced
- 1 pint cherry or grape tomatoes, halved
- 1/2 red onion, diced
- 1/4 cup fresh parsley, chopped
- 2 tbsp fresh mint, chopped
- Juice of 1 lemon
- 2 tbsp olive oil
- 1 tbsp red wine vinegar
- 1 garlic clove, minced
- 1 tsp dried oregano
- Salt and pepper to taste
- Crumbled feta cheese (optional)

Instructions:
1. In a large bowl, combine the chickpeas, diced cucumber, halved tomatoes, red onion, parsley and mint.

2. In a small bowl, whisk together the lemon juice, olive oil, red wine vinegar, garlic, oregano and a pinch each of salt and pepper.

3. Pour the lemon dressing over the chickpea salad and toss gently to coat.

4. Taste and adjust seasoning as needed, adding more lemon juice for brightness or oil for richness.

5. If desired, fold in some crumbled feta cheese.

6. Let the salad marinate for at least 30 minutes before serving to allow flavors to blend.

7. Serve chilled or at room temperature. Can be made a few hours in advance.

This fresh, vibrant chickpea salad is high in protein and fiber from the chickpeas and veggies. The herbs add great flavor along with the zesty lemon dressing. It makes a wonderful light main course salad or a tasty side salad for grilled proteins. You can add other salad veggies you have on hand as well. It's a versatile, nutritious vegetarian dish perfect for spring and summer.

11. Baked cod with roasted Brussels sprouts

Ingredients:
- 1 lb cod fillets
- 2 tbsp olive oil, divided
- 1 lemon, zested and juiced
- 1 tsp dried thyme
- Salt and pepper to taste
- 1 lb Brussels sprouts, trimmed and halved
- 3 cloves garlic, minced
- 1 tbsp balsamic vinegar
- 2 tbsp grated parmesan

Instructions:

1. Preheat oven to 400°F. Line a baking sheet with foil or parchment paper.

2. Pat the cod fillets dry and place them on the baking sheet. Drizzle with 1 tbsp olive oil, lemon zest, thyme, and season with salt and pepper.

3. On another baking sheet, toss the halved Brussels sprouts with remaining 1 tbsp olive oil, minced garlic, balsamic vinegar and salt and pepper. Spread out in a single layer.

4. Place both baking sheets in the preheated oven. Roast the Brussels sprouts for 20-25 minutes, shaking the pan halfway, until sprouts are browned and tender.

5. Bake the cod for 12-15 minutes, until opaque in the center and flakes easily with a fork.

6. Remove both from the oven. Transfer roasted Brussels sprouts to a bowl and toss with the parmesan.

7. Squeeze fresh lemon juice over the baked cod fillets.

8. Serve the cod warm with the roasted parmesan brussels sprouts on the side.

This baked cod and roasted brussels sprouts dish makes a healthy, flavorful meal with bright lemon notes. The cod stays tender while roasting gives the brussels sprouts a wonderful crispy, caramelized texture. You can use the same oven to efficiently cook both components. Feel free to adjust baking times as needed for desired doneness.

12. Brown rice pilaf with roasted vegetables

Ingredients:
- 1 cup brown rice
- 2 cups low-sodium vegetable or chicken broth
- 1 tbsp olive oil
- 1 shallot, diced
- 2 cloves garlic, minced
- 1 tsp dried thyme
- 1/4 cup dry white wine (optional)

- 1 cup diced carrots
- 1 cup diced zucchini
- 1 red bell pepper, diced
- 1 cup cauliflower florets
- 2 tbsp olive oil
- Salt and pepper to taste
- 2 tbsp chopped fresh parsley

Instructions:

1. Preheat oven to 425°F. Line a baking sheet with parchment paper.

2. In a saucepan, bring the broth to a simmer. Add the brown rice, cover and reduce heat to low. Simmer for 40-45 minutes until rice is tender.

3. Meanwhile, heat 1 tbsp olive oil in a skillet over medium heat. Add the shallot and cook 2 minutes until translucent.

4. Add the garlic and thyme and cook 1 minute until fragrant.

5. Deglaze the pan with the white wine if using, scraping up any browned bits.

6. Remove from heat and set aside.

7. On the prepared baking sheet, toss the diced carrots, zucchini, bell pepper and cauliflower with 2 tbsp olive oil. Season with salt and pepper.

8. Roast for 20-25 minutes, tossing halfway, until vegetables are tender and browned.

9. Once rice is cooked, fluff with a fork and stir in the shallot mixture and roasted vegetables. Garnish with chopped fresh parsley.

This hearty vegetarian pilaf combines protein and fiber from the brown rice with an assortment of roasted vegetables. The shallot, garlic and thyme add great flavor. You can use any combination of your favorite roasted veggies like Brussels sprouts, butternut squash or asparagus. It makes a nutritious vegetarian main or an excellent side dish.

13. Turkey chili with kidney beans

Ingredients:
- 1 tbsp olive oil
- 1 lb ground turkey
- 1 onion, diced
- 3 cloves garlic, minced
- 2 tbsp chili powder
- 2 tsp ground cumin
- 1 tsp dried oregano
- 1/4 tsp cayenne pepper (or to taste)
- 1 (28oz) can crushed tomatoes
- 2 (15oz) cans kidney beans, drained and rinsed
- 2 cups chicken or turkey broth
- Salt and pepper to taste
- Toppings: shredded cheese, diced avocado, sour cream, etc.

Instructions:
1. In a large pot or dutch oven, heat the olive oil over medium-high heat. Add the ground turkey and cook until no longer pink, 5-7 minutes, making sure to crumble the turkey as it cooks. Drain any excess fat.

2. Add the onion to the pot and cook for 2-3 minutes until translucent. Add the garlic and cook for 1 minute until fragrant.

3. Stir in the chili powder, cumin, oregano, cayenne, and a pinch each of salt and pepper. Toast the spices for 1 minute.

4. Pour in the crushed tomatoes, kidney beans, and broth. Bring to a boil.

5. Reduce heat and let the chili simmer for 20-30 minutes, until slightly thickened.

6. Taste and adjust seasoning as needed, adding more salt/pepper or spices.

7. Serve the chili warm topped with shredded cheese, avocado, sour cream, etc. if desired.

This turkey chili is protein-packed, flavorful, and lower in fat than beef chili. The kidney beans make it hearty and filling. You can use ground chicken instead of turkey if preferred. Adjust the spice level to taste by increasing or decreasing the cayenne. Optionally, add a splash of broth or water to thin out the chili. It makes great leftovers and freezes well too.

14. Cauliflower rice stir-fry with tofu

Ingredients:
- 1 head cauliflower, riced
(or 4 cups cauliflower rice)
- 14 oz extra-firm tofu, drained,
pressed and cubed
- 2 tbsp soy sauce or tamari, divided
- 2 tbsp rice vinegar
- 1 tbsp sesame oil
- 2 tsp cornstarch
- 2 tbsp vegetable oil
- 1 red bell pepper, sliced
- 4 oz mushrooms, sliced
- 2 garlic cloves, minced
- 1 tbsp grated fresh ginger
- 4 green onions, sliced, whites
and greens separated
- 1 cup frozen peas and carrots
- Salt and pepper to taste

Instructions:

1. If using a whole head of cauliflower, remove the core and coarsely chop into florets. Place in a food processor and pulse until cauliflower has a rice-like texture. You can also use pre-riced cauliflower.

2. Toss the cubed tofu with 1 tbsp soy sauce or tamari and let marinate briefly.

3. In a small bowl, whisk the vinegar, remaining 1 tbsp soy sauce, sesame oil, and cornstarch.

4. Heat vegetable oil in a large skillet or wok over high heat. Add the marinated tofu and stir-fry for 2-3 minutes until lightly browned on the outside. Transfer to a plate.

5. In the same skillet, add the bell pepper and mushrooms. Stir-fry for 2 minutes.

6. Add the garlic, ginger, and white parts of the green onions. Stir-fry for 1 minute until fragrant.

7. Add the cauliflower rice and stir-fry for 2-3 minutes until beginning to soften slightly.

8. Whisk the soy sauce mixture again to incorporate the cornstarch, then pour into the skillet and toss to coat the veggies and cauliflower.

9. Add back the tofu and the frozen peas/carrots. Continue stirring for 1-2 minutes until sauce thickens.

10. Remove from heat and stir in the green parts of the onions. Season with salt and pepper. Serve the cauliflower rice stir-fry immediately while hot.

This veggie-packed stir-fry is a healthy, low-carb alternative to rice, using riced cauliflower instead. The tofu adds plant-based protein. Feel free to mix up the vegetables based on your preferences or what you have on hand. Adjust soy sauce amounts to taste as well.

15. Greek salad with grilled chicken

Ingredients:
- 4 boneless, skinless chicken breasts
- 2 tbsp olive oil, plus more for grilling
- 1 tbsp lemon juice
- 2 cloves garlic, minced
- 1 tsp dried oregano
- Salt and pepper
- 1 romaine heart, chopped
- 1 cucumber, diced
- 1 cup cherry tomatoes, halved
- 1/2 red onion, thinly sliced
- 1/2 cup Kalamata olives, pitted
- 4 oz feta cheese, crumbled

Greek Dressing:
- 1/4 cup olive oil
- 2 tbsp red wine vinegar
- 1 tbsp lemon juice
- 2 tsp dried oregano
- 1 garlic clove, minced
- Salt and pepper to taste

Instructions:

1. In a shallow dish, combine 2 tbsp olive oil, 1 tbsp lemon juice, garlic, oregano, and salt and pepper. Add chicken breasts and turn to coat. Let marinate for 30 minutes at room temperature.

2. Make the dressing by whisking together the olive oil, vinegar, lemon juice, oregano, garlic, and salt and pepper in a small bowl or jar.

3. Preheat grill or grill pan to medium-high heat and brush grates with oil.

4. Grill the chicken for 6-8 minutes per side until cooked through. Allow to rest 5 minutes then slice.

5. In a large salad bowl, toss together the chopped romaine, cucumber, cherry tomatoes, red onion, olives, and feta cheese. Drizzle desired amount of Greek dressing over the salad mixture and toss to coat.

6. Top the salad with the sliced grilled chicken. Serve the Greek salad immediately while the chicken is hot, with any extra dressing on the side.

This fresh and flavorful salad combines classic Greek salad ingredients like romaine, tomatoes, cucumber, feta, and olives with grilled chicken for added protein. The tangy Greek vinaigrette perfectly complements the salad. It's healthy, delicious, and great for summer meals. You can cook the chicken on outdoor or indoor grill.

16. Roasted vegetable and chickpea Buddha bowl

Ingredients:
- 1 sweet potato, diced
- 1 bell pepper, diced
- 1/2 red onion, sliced
- 8 oz brussels sprouts, halved
- 2 tbsp olive oil
- 1 tsp cumin
- Salt and pepper
- 1 (15oz) can chickpeas, drained and rinsed
- 1 cup cooked quinoa or brown rice
- 1 avocado, diced
- 1/4 cup crumbled feta or goat cheese
- 2 tbsp sunflower or pumpkin seeds

Tahini Dressing:
- 1/4 cup tahini
- 2 tbsp lemon juice
- 2 tbsp olive oil
- 1 garlic clove, minced
- 2-4 tbsp water to thin
- Salt and pepper to taste

Instructions:

1. Preheat oven to 400°F. On a baking sheet, toss the diced sweet potato, bell pepper, red onion and brussels sprouts with 2 tbsp olive oil, cumin, salt and pepper.

2. Roast for 25-30 minutes, tossing halfway, until vegetables are tender and browned.

3. Remove from oven and toss roasted veggies with the drained, rinsed chickpeas.

4. Make the tahini dressing by whisking together the tahini, lemon juice, olive oil, garlic, and enough water to reach a drizzlable consistency. Season with salt and pepper.

5. Assemble the Buddha bowls by dividing the cooked quinoa or rice between bowls. Top with the roasted veggie/chickpea mixture.

6. Garnish with diced avocado, crumbled cheese, sunflower seeds and a drizzle of the tahini dressing.

These veggie-packed Buddha bowls make a healthy, plant-based meal full of different textures and flavors. The roasted veggies pair beautifully with the chickpeas, whole grains, creamy avocado and tangy tahini sauce. You can customize the bowls with your choice of roasted veggies too. Great for meal prep!

17. Sardine salad with mixed greens

Ingredients:
- 5 oz can sardines in olive oil, drained
- 6 cups mixed greens
 (romaine, arugula, spinach)
- 1/2 cup cherry tomatoes, halved
- 1/4 red onion, thinly sliced
- 2 hard-boiled eggs, sliced
- 1/4 cup Kalamata olives, pitted and halved
- 2 tbsp capers, drained
- 2 tbsp fresh parsley, chopped

Lemon Vinaigrette:
- 2 tbsp olive oil
- 2 tbsp lemon juice
- 1 tsp Dijon mustard
- 1 garlic clove, minced
- Salt and pepper to taste

Instructions:

1. Make the vinaigrette by whisking together the olive oil, lemon juice, mustard, garlic, and salt and pepper in a bowl or jar.

2. In a large salad bowl, add the mixed greens, cherry tomatoes, sliced red onion, hard-boiled egg slices, olives, and capers.

3. Break up the sardines and add them to the salad bowl along with any olive oil from the can.

4. Drizzle the desired amount of lemon vinaigrette over the salad and toss gently to coat.

5. Let the salad sit for 5 minutes to allow the flavors to blend.

6. Garnish with chopped fresh parsley before serving.

This protein-packed salad combines nutrient-dense sardines with fresh vegetables, eggs, olives and capers for a variety of flavors and textures. The bright lemon vinaigrette complements the briny sardines perfectly. Sardines are an excellent source of omega-3s, vitamin D and calcium. Serve as a light main course or divide into side salad portions.

18. Eggplant lasagna with ground turkey

Ingredients:
- 2 large eggplants, sliced into 1/4 inch rounds
- Salt for sweating eggplant
- 1 tbsp olive oil
- 1 onion, diced
- 3 cloves garlic, minced
- 1 lb ground turkey
- 2 cups marinara sauce
- 1 cup low-fat ricotta cheese
- 1 egg
- 1/4 cup grated parmesan
- 1 tsp dried basil
- Salt and pepper to taste
- 9 oz shredded part-skim mozzarella cheese
- Chopped parsley for garnish

Instructions:

1. Lay the eggplant slices on paper towels and sprinkle with salt. Let sit for 30 minutes to draw out moisture, then pat dry.

2. Brush or spray the eggplant slices with olive oil on both sides. Grill, bake at 400°F, or air fry until lightly browned.

3. In a skillet, cook the onion and garlic in olive oil over medium heat until soft. Add the ground turkey and cook until browned, 5-7 minutes. Drain excess fat.

4. In a bowl, mix the ricotta, egg, parmesan, basil and salt/pepper.

5. In a 9x13 baking dish, spread 1/2 cup marinara sauce on the bottom. Layer with 1/3 of the eggplant slices, 1/2 the turkey mixture, 1/2 the ricotta mixture, and 1/3 of the mozzarella. Repeat layers ending with mozzarella.

6. Cover and bake at 375°F for 30 minutes. Uncover and bake 15 more minutes until hot and bubbly. Let stand 10 minutes before serving. Garnish with parsley.

This has anti-inflammatory eggplant, lean turkey instead of beef, and part-skim dairy. The marinara provides nutrients while keeping it lower in fat and calories than a traditional lasagna. Enjoy!

19. Beet and kale salad with goat cheese

Ingredients:
- 4 medium beets, roasted and diced
- 1 large bunch kale, stemmed and chopped into bite-sized pieces (about 6 cups)
- 1/2 cup crumbled goat cheese
- 1/4 cup dried cranberries
- 1/4 cup toasted pecan halves
- 2 tbsp olive oil
- 2 tbsp balsamic vinegar
- 1 tsp Dijon mustard
- 1 garlic clove, minced
- Salt and pepper to taste

Instructions:

1. Roast the beets: Preheat oven to 400°F. Wrap beets in foil and roast for 50-60 minutes until fork tender. Allow to cool, then peel and dice into 1/2 inch cubes.

2. Make the dressing: In a small bowl, whisk together the olive oil, balsamic vinegar, Dijon mustard, garlic and a pinch each of salt and pepper.

3. In a large bowl, toss the chopped kale with about half of the dressing. Use your hands to massage the dressing into the kale to help tenderize the leaves.

4. Add the roasted beets, dried cranberries, pecan halves and goat cheese crumbles to the kale.

5. Drizzle the remaining dressing over top and toss gently to combine.

6. Let the salad sit for 5-10 minutes to allow the flavors to meld together.

7. Taste and adjust seasoning as needed, adding more salt, pepper, vinegar, etc. if desired.

8. Serve immediately while the salad is fresh and the flavors are vibrant.

This salad provides a great mix of nutrients with the antioxidant-rich beets, vitamin K and fiber from the kale, protein from the goat cheese, and healthy fats from the olive oil and pecans. The tart cranberries and tangy balsamic dressing add a nice bright pop of flavor too. Enjoy!

20. Chicken and vegetable kebabs with quinoa

Ingredients:
- 1 lb boneless, skinless chicken breasts,
cut into 1-inch cubes
- 2 bell peppers (colors of your choice),
cut into 1-inch pieces
- 1 red onion, cut into 1-inch pieces
- 1 zucchini, sliced into 1/2-inch thick rounds
- 8 oz mushrooms,
left whole if small or halved if large
- 2 tbsp olive oil
- 2 tsp Italian seasoning
- Salt and pepper to taste
- 1 cup quinoa
- 2 cups vegetable or chicken broth

For the Marinade:
- 1/4 cup olive oil
- 3 tbsp lemon juice
- 2 garlic cloves, minced
- 1 tsp dried oregano
- 1/2 tsp salt
- 1/4 tsp pepper

Instructions:

1. Make the marinade by whisking together the olive oil, lemon juice, garlic, oregano, salt and pepper. Add the cubed chicken and toss to coat. Cover and marinate for 30 minutes to 1 hour.

2. Cook the quinoa according to package instructions, substituting broth for water to add more flavor. Fluff with a fork when done.

3. Preheat grill or grill pan to medium-high heat. Thread the marinated chicken, bell peppers, onions, zucchini and mushrooms onto skewers in an alternating pattern.

4. In a small bowl, toss the skewered vegetables with 2 tbsp olive oil, Italian seasoning, salt and pepper.

5. Grill the kebabs for 12-15 minutes, turning occasionally, until the chicken is cooked through and the vegetables are tender.

6. Serve the kebabs over a bed of the cooked quinoa. Garnish with fresh parsley or basil if desired.

This meal provides lean protein from the chicken, fiber and nutrients from the grilled veggies, and the quinoa adds whole grains, protein and texture. The lemon marinade adds amazing flavor. You can mix up the veggie variety based on your preferences too. Enjoy!

21. Lentil and spinach salad with lemon vinaigrette

Ingredients:
- 1 cup dried green or brown lentils, rinsed
- 1 bay leaf
- 5 oz baby spinach
- 1 cup cherry tomatoes, halved
- 1/2 English cucumber, diced
- 1/4 red onion, thinly sliced
- 1/4 cup crumbled feta cheese

Lemon Vinaigrette:
- 1/4 cup olive oil
- 2 tbsp lemon juice
- 1 garlic clove, minced
- 1 tsp Dijon mustard
- 1 tsp honey
- Salt and pepper to taste

Instructions:

1. Add the lentils and bay leaf to a saucepan and cover with 2 inches of water or broth. Bring to a boil, then reduce heat and simmer for 20-25 minutes until lentils are tender but still hold their shape. Drain and discard bay leaf.

2. Transfer warm lentils to a large bowl and toss with the baby spinach to lightly wilt the greens.

3. In a small bowl or jar, whisk together all the vinaigrette ingredients until emulsified.

4. Add the cherry tomatoes, cucumber, red onion and feta to the lentil-spinach mixture. Pour the vinaigrette over top and toss gently to combine.

5. Taste and adjust seasoning as needed, adding more lemon, salt, pepper, etc.

6. Let sit for 10-15 minutes to allow flavors to meld before serving at room temperature or chilled.

This salad provides a great mix of plant protein from the lentils, greens from the spinach, and a variety of other veggies. The lemon vinaigrette adds fresh, bright flavor. It makes a filling vegetarian meal on its own or a tasty side salad. You can also add grilled chicken or shrimp if you want to boost the protein content further.

22. Baked halibut with asparagus

Ingredients:
- 4 (6oz) halibut fillets
- 1 lb asparagus, trimmed
- 2 tbsp olive oil, divided
- Salt and pepper to taste
- 1 lemon, sliced into rounds
- 2 cloves garlic, minced
- 1 tsp dried thyme
- 2 tbsp white wine or vegetable broth
- 2 tbsp unsalted butter
- 2 tbsp fresh parsley, chopped
- Lemon wedges for serving

Instructions:
1. Preheat oven to 400°F. Line a baking sheet with foil or parchment paper.

2. Arrange the asparagus in a single layer on the prepared baking sheet. Drizzle with 1 tbsp olive oil and season with salt and pepper.

3. Push the asparagus to one side of the baking sheet and arrange the halibut fillets on the other side.

4. Drizzle the halibut with the remaining 1 tbsp olive oil and season with salt and pepper. Top each fillet with a slice or two of lemon.

5. In a small bowl, combine the minced garlic, dried thyme, and white wine/broth. Pour the mixture over the halibut and asparagus.

6. Bake for 12-15 minutes, until the fish is opaque and flakes easily with a fork and the asparagus is tender.

7. Remove from oven and top the halibut with pats of butter to allow it to melt over top.

8. Garnish the halibut and asparagus with the chopped fresh parsley.

9. Serve immediately with lemon wedges for squeezing over top.

This dish is not only delicious but also very nutritious. The halibut provides lean protein and heart-healthy omega-3 fatty acids. The asparagus is rich in fiber, vitamins and antioxidants. The olive oil, butter, garlic, thyme and lemon add fantastic flavor.

23. Quinoa tabbouleh with grilled shrimp

Ingredients:
- 1 cup quinoa
- 2 cups vegetable or chicken broth
- 1 cup finely chopped parsley
- 1/2 cup finely chopped mint
- 1/2 cup finely diced tomato
- 1/2 cup finely diced cucumber
- 1/4 cup finely sliced green onions
- 3 tbsp lemon juice
- 2 tbsp olive oil
- 1 tsp sumac (or lemon zest)
- Salt and pepper to taste
- 1 lb shrimp, peeled and deveined
- 1 tbsp olive oil
- 1 tsp paprika
- 1 garlic clove, minced

Instructions:

1. Cook the quinoa according to package instructions, substituting broth for water. Fluff with a fork and let cool completely.

2. In a large bowl, combine the cooled quinoa, parsley, mint, tomato, cucumber, green onions, lemon juice, olive oil, and sumac. Season with salt and pepper to taste.

3. Toss the shrimp with 1 tbsp olive oil, paprika, garlic and a pinch of salt and pepper.

4. Heat a grill or grill pan over medium-high heat. Grill the shrimp for 2-3 minutes per side until opaque and cooked through.

5. Add the grilled shrimp to the quinoa tabbouleh and gently toss to combine. Taste and adjust seasoning if needed, adding more lemon juice, olive oil, salt or pepper.

6. Serve the tabbouleh at room temperature or chilled. Garnish with extra parsley or mint if desired.

This dish combines the fresh flavors of traditional tabbouleh with protein-packed quinoa and grilled shrimp. It's light yet satisfying, perfect for a summer meal. The quinoa provides fiber and plant-based protein. The herbs and lemon add vibrancy. And the grilled shrimp gives you lean protein with a nice charred flavor. You can adjust the proportions of the ingredients to your taste preferences as well.

24. Stuffed acorn squash with wild rice and cranberries

Ingredients:
- 2 medium acorn squash, halved and seeded
- 2 tbsp olive oil, divided
- Salt and pepper to taste
- 1 cup uncooked wild rice blend
- 2 cups vegetable or chicken broth
- 1/4 cup dried cranberries
- 1/4 cup toasted pecans, chopped
- 2 green onions, sliced
- 2 tbsp fresh parsley, chopped
- 2 tbsp butter
- 2 cloves garlic, minced
- 1/4 cup grated parmesan cheese

Instructions:

1. Preheat oven to 400°F. Brush the acorn squash cavities with 1 tbsp olive oil and sprinkle with salt and pepper. Place cut-side down on a baking sheet and roast for 30 minutes.

2. Meanwhile, cook the wild rice blend according to package instructions, substituting broth for water.

3. In a skillet, heat the remaining 1 tbsp olive oil over medium heat. Add the garlic and sauté for 1 minute until fragrant.

4. Remove cooked wild rice from heat and stir in the cranberries, pecans, green onions, parsley, butter, garlic, and parmesan. Season with salt and pepper.

5. Remove squash from oven and carefully flip over cut-side up. Fill cavities evenly with the wild rice stuffing mixture.

6. Return to oven and bake for 15-20 more minutes until squash is very tender when pierced with a fork.

7. Let cool slightly before serving. The stuffing and squash can be served directly in the squash halves or scooped out.

This makes a wonderfully nutritious vegetarian main dish. The wild rice blend provides fiber, protein and nutrients. The cranberries add sweetness and the pecans give a crunch. Roasting the acorn squash allows it to get soft and sweet. You get lots of great fall flavors in one healthy package! Delicious on its own or with a side salad.

25. Spaghetti squash with turkey meatballs and marinara sauce

Ingredients:
For the Spaghetti Squash:
- 1 large spaghetti squash
- 2 tbsp olive oil
- Salt and pepper to taste

For the Marinara Sauce:
- 1 tbsp olive oil
- 1 onion, diced
- 3 garlic cloves, minced
- 1 (28oz) can crushed tomatoes
- 1 tsp dried basil
- Salt and pepper to taste

For the Turkey Meatballs:
- 1 lb ground turkey
- 1 egg
- 1/4 cup breadcrumbs
- 1/4 cup grated parmesan
- 2 garlic cloves, minced
- 1 tsp dried basil
- 1 tsp dried parsley
- Salt and pepper to taste

Instructions:

1. Roast the spaghetti squash: Preheat oven to 400°F. Cut squash in half lengthwise and scoop out seeds. Rub the flesh with 2 tbsp olive oil and season with salt and pepper. Place cut-side down on a baking sheet and roast for 40-50 minutes until very tender.

2. Make the turkey meatballs: In a bowl, mix together the turkey, egg, breadcrumbs, parmesan, garlic, basil, parsley, and salt and pepper. Roll into 1-inch meatballs and place on a greased baking sheet. Bake at 400°F for 15-18 minutes until cooked through.

3. Make the marinara sauce: In a saucepan, sauté the onion and garlic in olive oil over medium heat for 2-3 minutes until fragrant. Add the crushed tomatoes, basil, and salt and pepper. Simmer for 10-15 minutes, stirring occasionally.

4. Once squash is done, use a fork to scrape out the flesh into strands, transferring it to a serving dish.

5. Add the cooked turkey meatballs to the marinara sauce and gently toss to coat. Top the spaghetti squash strands with the meatball marinara sauce. Garnish with extra parmesan and parsley if desired. Serve hot.

This lightened up version gives you all the flavor of spaghetti and meatballs, but in a more nutritious way! The spaghetti squash provides fiber, while the turkey meatballs are leaner than beef. Enjoy this delicious baked "pasta" dish!

26. Tofu and vegetable stir-fry with brown rice

Ingredients:
- 1 cup brown rice
- 1 (14 oz) package extra-firm tofu, drained and cubed
- 2 tbsp sesame oil, divided
- 2 cloves garlic, minced
- 1 tbsp grated fresh ginger
- 1 cup broccoli florets
- 1 red bell pepper, sliced
- 1 cup snap peas
- 1 cup shredded cabbage or coleslaw mix
- 3 green onions, sliced
- 3 tbsp low-sodium soy sauce
- 1 tbsp rice vinegar
- 1 tsp sriracha or chili garlic sauce (optional)
- 1 tsp sesame seeds

Instructions:
1. Cook the brown rice according to package instructions. Keep warm.

2. Pat the tofu cubes dry with a paper towel and season with salt and pepper.

3. In a large skillet or wok, heat 1 tbsp sesame oil over medium-high heat. Add the tofu and cook for 5-7 minutes until lightly browned on a few sides. Transfer to a plate.

4. Add the remaining 1 tbsp sesame oil to the skillet along with the garlic and ginger. Cook for 1 minute until fragrant.

5. Add the broccoli, bell pepper, and snap peas. Stir-fry for 3-4 minutes.

6. Add the cabbage and green onions and continue to stir-fry for 2 more minutes.

7. In a small bowl, whisk together the soy sauce, rice vinegar, and sriracha (if using). Pour into the skillet and toss to coat everything.

8. Add the cooked tofu back to the skillet and gently toss everything together until heated through. Serve the stir-fry over the cooked brown rice. Garnish with sesame seeds.

This veggie-packed stir-fry is loaded with plant-based protein from the tofu and fiber from the brown rice and veggies. Using sesame oil adds nutty flavor. The soy sauce, ginger and sriracha (if you want heat) contribute savoriness. Feel free to substitute in other vegetables you enjoy as well. A quick and nutritious meatless meal!

27. Kale and white bean soup

Ingredients:
- 1 tbsp olive oil
- 1 onion, diced
- 3 cloves garlic, minced
- 4 cups vegetable or chicken broth
- 2 (15oz) cans cannellini or white beans, drained and rinsed
- 1 bunch kale, stems removed and leaves chopped
- 1 bay leaf
- 1 tsp dried thyme
- 1 tsp dried oregano
- Salt and pepper to taste
- Grated parmesan cheese for serving

Instructions:

1. In a large pot or dutch oven, heat the olive oil over medium heat. Add the onion and cook for 5 minutes until soft and translucent.

2. Add the garlic and cook for 1 more minute until fragrant.

3. Pour in the broth, beans, chopped kale, bay leaf, thyme, oregano. Season with salt and pepper to taste.

4. Bring the soup to a boil, then reduce heat and simmer for 15-20 minutes to allow flavors to meld.

5. Remove and discard the bay leaf. Use an immersion blender or regular blender to partially puree about 1/3 to 1/2 of the soup, leaving some beans and kale chunks intact for texture.

6. Return the partially blended soup to the pot and heat through. Adjust seasoning if needed. Serve the kale and white bean soup hot, garnished with grated parmesan cheese.

This nutritious soup packs in fiber, protein and antioxidants from the kale and beans. It's vegetarian but still hearty and filling. The parmesan adds a salty, savory element. You can use vegetable or chicken broth in this recipe. Other greens like spinach can be substituted for some of the kale if desired. Let it simmer longer for even more developed flavors.

This soup keeps well refrigerated for several days and can be frozen too. It makes a wonderfully healthy lunch or light dinner with some crusty bread on the side.

28. Grilled salmon with roasted sweet potatoes

Ingredients:
- 4 (6 oz) salmon fillets
- 2 tbsp olive oil, divided
- 1 tsp lemon pepper seasoning
- Salt and pepper to taste
- 3 medium sweet potatoes, peeled and cubed
- 1 tsp paprika
- 1 tsp garlic powder
- 2 tbsp chopped fresh parsley
- Lemon wedges for serving

Instructions:

1. Preheat grill to medium-high heat. Lightly oil the grill grates.

2. Brush the salmon fillets all over with 1 tbsp of the olive oil and season with lemon pepper, salt, and pepper.

3. On a baking sheet, toss the cubed sweet potatoes with the remaining 1 tbsp olive oil, paprika, garlic powder, and salt/pepper to taste.

4. Roast the sweet potatoes at 400°F for 25-30 minutes, stirring halfway, until tender and lightly browned.

5. Once the potatoes are almost done, grill the salmon for 4-6 minutes per side until opaque in the center and an internal temp of 145°F is reached.

6. Remove the roasted sweet potatoes from the oven and toss with the chopped fresh parsley.

7. Plate the grilled salmon fillets and roasted sweet potato cubes together. Serve with lemon wedges for squeezing over the fish.

This dish makes an excellent nutritious meal with lean protein from the salmon and vitamin/mineral-rich vegetables from the sweet potatoes. The grilled salmon provides beneficial omega-3 fatty acids, while the sweet potatoes offer fiber, vitamin A, and antioxidants.

Some tips:
- Let the salmon rest at room temperature for 15 minutes before grilling for more even cooking.Baste the salmon with lemon juice or a glaze partway through grilling if desired.
- Other seasoning blends like cajun or jerk can be substituted for the lemon pepper on the salmon.Top the roasted sweet potatoes with a sprinkle of feta or blue cheese for extra flavor.

This is an easy yet elegant and healthy main dish perfect for a weeknight or entertaining! Enjoy the fresh flavors of grilled fish and roasted veggies.

29. Mediterranean quinoa salad with feta cheese

Ingredients:

- 1 cup quinoa
- 2 cups vegetable or chicken broth
- 1 cup cherry tomatoes, halved
- 1 cucumber, diced
- 1/2 red onion, finely diced
- 1 bell pepper, diced
- 1/2 cup pitted kalamata olives, halved
- 1/2 cup crumbled feta cheese
- 1/4 cup chopped fresh parsley
- 2 tbsp chopped fresh mint
- Juice of 1 lemon
- 2 tbsp olive oil
- 2 cloves garlic, minced
- 1 tsp dried oregano
- Salt and pepper to taste

Instructions:

1. Cook the quinoa according to package instructions, using the broth instead of water. Fluff with a fork and let cool slightly.

2. In a large bowl, combine the cooked quinoa, cherry tomatoes, cucumber, red onion, bell pepper, olives, feta, parsley and mint.

3. In a small bowl, whisk together the lemon juice, olive oil, garlic, oregano, salt and pepper.

4. Pour the dressing over the quinoa salad and toss gently to combine all ingredients.

5. Taste and adjust seasoning as needed, adding more lemon juice for brightness or olive oil for richness.

6. Let the salad rest for at least 30 minutes before serving to allow flavors to meld. Can be served chilled or at room temperature.

This Mediterranean-inspired quinoa salad is loaded with fresh, bright flavors and textures. Quinoa makes a protein-packed base, while the tomatoes, cucumber, peppers and herbs lend vitamins and crunch. The feta adds a salty, tangy note that perfectly complements the lemony dressing.

You can make this salad a day in advance - it keeps very well refrigerated. It's perfect for meal prep lunches, potlucks or light summer dinners. Consider adding chickpeas or grilled chicken to make it even heartier. The fresh mint is key for tantalizing aroma, but you can sub extra parsley if needed. Enjoy this delightfully refreshing salad!

30. Baked chicken thighs with Brussels sprouts and carrots

Ingredients:
- 8 bone-in, skin-on chicken thighs
- 2 tbsp olive oil
- 1 tsp dried thyme
- 1 tsp dried rosemary
- 1 tbsp lemon juice
- 1 tbsp honey
- Salt and pepper to taste
- 1 lb Brussels sprouts, trimmed and halved
- 4 large carrots, peeled and cut into 1-inch pieces
- 2 cloves garlic, minced
- 2 tbsp butter, melted

Instructions:

1. Preheat oven to 400°F. Lightly grease a large baking sheet or dish.

2. Pat the chicken thighs dry and place them on the baking sheet. Drizzle with 1 tbsp of the olive oil and season both sides with thyme, rosemary, salt and pepper.

3. On the same baking sheet, toss the Brussels sprouts and carrots with the remaining 1 tbsp olive oil, minced garlic, salt and pepper.

4. Roast for 20 minutes. Remove from oven and use a spoon to toss the vegetables.

5. In a small bowl, whisk together the melted butter, lemon juice and honey.

6. Drizzle or brush the butter mixture over the chicken thighs and vegetables.

7. Return to the oven and roast for 20-25 more minutes, until chicken is cooked through (165°F internal temp) and vegetables are tender and caramelized.

8. Let chicken rest 5 minutes before serving with the roasted Brussels sprouts and carrots on the side.

This all-in-one sheet pan meal makes a complete and satisfying dinner with protein, veggies and flavor! Bone-in, skin-on chicken thighs stay deliciously juicy when roasted. The Brussels sprouts get crispy and browned, while the carrots turn sweet and tender.

The lemon-honey butter glaze caramelizes beautifully on everything, adding tons of rich flavor. You get hints of thyme, rosemary and garlic rounding it all out.

This recipe is also easy to adapt - try different veggie combos like potatoes, sweet potatoes, parsnips or cauliflower. The chicken can be swapped for drumsticks if desired too. For quick prep, everything gets tossed together and roasted on one pan for easy clean-up. Simple, nutritious and utterly delicious!

31. Lentil and vegetable stew

Ingredients:
- 1 cup dried green or brown lentils, rinsed
- 1 tbsp olive oil
- 1 onion, diced
- 3 carrots, peeled and sliced
- 3 stalks celery, sliced
- 4 cloves garlic, minced
- 1 tsp ground cumin
- 1 tsp dried thyme
- 1/4 tsp crushed red pepper flakes (optional for heat)
- 1 bay leaf
- 4 cups vegetable or chicken broth
- 1 (14.5 oz) can diced tomatoes
- 2 cups chopped kale or spinach
- Salt and pepper to taste
- Squeeze of lemon juice (optional)

Instructions:

1. In a large pot or dutch oven, heat the olive oil over medium-high heat. Add the onions and sauté for 2-3 minutes until translucent.

2. Add the carrots, celery, garlic, cumin, thyme, red pepper flakes (if using), and bay leaf. Cook for 2 more minutes.

3. Add the lentils, broth, and diced tomatoes with their juices. Bring to a boil.

4. Once boiling, reduce heat to low, cover and simmer for 20-25 minutes, until lentils are tender but still hold their shape.

5. Remove bay leaf. Stir in the chopped greens and let wilt for 2-3 minutes.

6. Season with salt, pepper, and a squeeze of lemon juice if desired.

7. Serve hot, optionally with crusty bread on the side.

This hearty stew is packed with plant-based protein from the lentils as well as plenty of vegetables. It makes great leftovers too! You can adjust vegetables based on what you have on hand.

32. Zucchini noodles with turkey bolognese sauce

Ingredients:
- 4 medium zucchinis
- 1 tbsp olive oil
- 1 lb ground turkey
- 1 onion, diced
- 3 cloves garlic, minced
- 1 carrot, peeled and grated
- 2 stalks celery, diced
- 1 (28oz) can crushed tomatoes
- 1⁄4 cup red wine (optional)
- 2 tsp dried basil
- 1 tsp dried oregano
- 1⁄4 tsp red pepper flakes
- Salt and pepper to taste
- 1⁄4 cup grated parmesan, plus more for serving
- Chopped parsley for garnish

Instructions:

1. Use a spiralizer or julienne peeler to cut the zucchinis into noodle shapes. Set aside.

2. In a large skillet or saucepan, heat the olive oil over medium-high heat. Add the ground turkey and cook until browned and crumbled, 5-7 minutes.

3. Add the onions, garlic, carrots and celery. Cook for 3-4 more minutes until softened.

4. Pour in the crushed tomatoes and red wine if using. Add the basil, oregano, red pepper flakes and season with salt and pepper to taste.

5. Bring the sauce to a simmer and let cook for 15-20 minutes, until slightly thickened.

6. Add the zucchini noodles and grated parmesan to the sauce and toss to combine. Cook for 2-3 minutes until the zucchini noodles are slightly softened but still crisp.

7. Remove from heat and garnish with more grated parmesan and chopped parsley before serving.

This makes a lighter take on spaghetti bolognese by using zucchini noodles instead of regular pasta. The turkey bolognese sauce is hearty and flavorful while letting the zucchini noodles shine. It's a delicious low-carb meal!

33. Black bean and corn salad with avocado

Ingredients:
- 1 (15 oz) can black beans, drained and rinsed
- 1 cup frozen corn kernels, thawed
- 1 avocado, diced
- 1/2 red onion, finely diced
- 1 jalapeno, seeded and finely chopped
- 1/4 cup chopped fresh cilantro
- 2 tbsp lime juice
- 2 tbsp olive oil
- 1 tsp ground cumin
- Salt and pepper to taste

Instructions:
1. In a large bowl, combine the drained black beans, thawed corn kernels, diced avocado, diced red onion, chopped jalapeno, and chopped cilantro.

2. In a small bowl, whisk together the lime juice, olive oil, cumin, and a pinch each of salt and pepper.

3. Pour the lime juice dressing over the bean and vegetable mixture. Toss gently to coat everything evenly.

4. Taste and adjust seasoning as needed, adding more salt, pepper, lime, or cumin to your taste preferences.

5. Optionally let the salad marinate for 30 minutes to allow flavors to blend before serving.

6. When ready to serve, give it one last gentle toss and transfer to a serving bowl or plate.

This vibrant black bean and corn salad is wonderfully fresh and flavorful. The avocado adds a rich, creamy element while the jalapeno provides a kick of heat. It makes a great side dish but is hearty enough to enjoy as a vegetarian entree salad as well. Feel free to add extras like diced tomato, crumbled feta or queso fresco.

34. Broiled mackerel with steamed green beans

Ingredients:
- 4 mackerel fillets
- 2 tbsp olive oil
- 1 lemon, sliced into wedges
- Salt and pepper to taste
- 1 lb fresh green beans, trimmed
- 1 tbsp butter or olive oil

For the mackerel:
1. Preheat your oven's broiler and position a rack 6 inches from the heating element. Line a baking sheet with foil.

2. Pat the mackerel fillets dry and place them skin-side down on the prepared baking sheet. Brush them with olive oil and season with salt and pepper.

3. Broil for 6-8 minutes, keeping a close eye to prevent burning, until the fish is opaque and flakes easily with a fork.

4. Squeeze fresh lemon juice over the top of the broiled mackerel fillets.

For the green beans:
1. Prepare an ice bath by filling a bowl with ice water. Set aside.

2. Bring a pot of salted water to a boil. Add the trimmed green beans and blanch for 3-4 minutes until bright green and crisp-tender.

3. Immediately drain the beans and plunge them into the ice bath to stop the cooking.

4. Once cooled, drain the beans and transfer to a bowl. Toss with the butter or olive oil and season with salt and pepper to taste.

To serve:
Transfer the broiled mackerel fillets to plates and serve with the steamed green beans on the side. The broiled fish gets nice and crispy while staying incredibly moist and flaky inside. The bright lemon pairs beautifully with the rich mackerel. Enjoy!

35. Quinoa and black bean stuffed peppers

Ingredients:
- 6 bell peppers, any color, tops cut off and seeds/membranes removed
- 1 cup quinoa, rinsed
- 2 cups vegetable or chicken broth
- 1 (15 oz) can black beans, drained and rinsed
- 1 cup corn kernels (fresh or frozen)
- 1/2 cup salsa
- 1 tsp cumin
- 1 tsp chili powder
- 1/2 tsp garlic powder
- 1/4 tsp cayenne pepper (optional)
- 1 cup shredded cheese (cheddar, monterey jack, etc)
- 2 tbsp chopped cilantro
- Salt and pepper to taste

Instructions:
1. Preheat oven to 375°F. Lightly grease a baking dish and place hollowed out pepper halves cut-side up in the dish.

2. In a saucepan, combine the quinoa and broth. Bring to a boil, then reduce heat to low, cover and simmer for 15-20 minutes until quinoa is fluffy.

3. In a bowl, mix together the cooked quinoa, black beans, corn, salsa, cumin, chili powder, garlic powder, cayenne (if using) and salt/pepper to taste.

4. Fill each pepper half evenly with the quinoa and bean mixture. Top with shredded cheese.

5. Pour a small amount of water or broth into the bottom of the baking dish. Cover with foil.

6. Bake for 30 minutes. Remove foil and bake 10-15 minutes more until peppers are tender and filling is heated through.

7. Remove from oven and let cool slightly. Garnish with chopped cilantro before serving.

These hearty vegetarian stuffed peppers make a flavorful and nutritious meal. The quinoa adds protein while the black beans, corn and salsa provide lots of southwestern flair. You can adjust the spices to your heat preference. Delicious served with extras like guacamole, sour cream or hot sauce on the side.

36. Grilled vegetable platter with hummus

For the Grilled Veggies:
- 1 zucchini, sliced into 1/4 inch rounds
- 1 yellow squash, sliced into 1/4 inch rounds
- 1 red bell pepper, seeded and quartered
- 1 yellow or orange bell pepper,
seeded and quartered
- 1 red onion, sliced into 1/2 inch rounds
- 8oz mushrooms, stems removed
- 1 eggplant, sliced into 1/2 inch rounds
- Olive oil
- Salt and pepper

For the Hummus:
- 1 (15oz) can chickpeas, drained
with liquid reserved
- 1/4 cup tahini
- 2 cloves garlic
- 1/4 cup lemon juice
- 2 tbsp olive oil
- 1 tsp ground cumin
- Salt to taste

Instructions:

1. Preheat grill to medium-high heat. Brush or toss the sliced vegetables with olive oil and season with salt and pepper.

2. Grill the vegetables in batches until tender and slightly charred, about 2-4 minutes per side depending on thickness. Transfer to a platter as done.

3. To make the hummus, add the chickpeas, tahini, garlic, lemon juice, olive oil and cumin to a food processor or blender. Blend until smooth, adding reserved chickpea liquid as needed to reach desired consistency. Season with salt to taste.

4. Transfer the hummus to a bowl and add to the platter with the grilled veggies.

5. Garnish the platter with fresh parsley, lemon wedges, feta cheese crumbles or toasted pine nuts if desired.

6. Serve the grilled vegetable platter with pita bread, pita chips or fresh veggies for dipping into the hummus.

This makes a beautiful, colorful platter that is perfect for entertaining or to enjoy as a light meatless meal. The smoky grilled veggies pair delightfully with the creamy, protein-packed hummus dip. It's a healthy yet satisfying dish that celebrates the bounty of seasonal vegetables.

37. Chicken and vegetable curry with quinoa

Ingredients:
- 1 red bell pepper, cut into strips
- 2 carrots, peeled and sliced
- 1 cup cauliflower florets
- 1 (14 oz) can diced tomatoes
- 1 (14 oz) can coconut milk
- 1 cup quinoa, rinsed
- 1/4 cup chopped cilantro
- Lime wedges for serving

- 1 lb boneless, skinless chicken breasts, cut into 1-inch cubes
- 1 tbsp curry powder
- 1 tsp ground cumin
- 1/4 tsp cayenne pepper (or to taste)
- 1/2 tsp salt
- 2 tbsp olive oil
- 1 onion, diced
- 3 cloves garlic, minced
- 1 tbsp freshly grated ginger

Instructions:

1. In a bowl, toss the cubed chicken with the curry powder, cumin, cayenne and salt until evenly coated.

2. In a large skillet or pot, heat the olive oil over medium-high heat. Add the chicken and cook for 4-5 minutes until browned but not cooked through. Transfer chicken to a plate.

3. In the same skillet, add the onions and sauté for 2 minutes until translucent. Add the garlic and ginger and cook for 1 minute until fragrant.

4. Add the bell pepper, carrots, cauliflower, diced tomatoes with juices and coconut milk. Bring to a simmer.

5. Return the partially cooked chicken and any accumulated juices to the skillet. Simmer for 10-12 minutes until chicken is cooked through and vegetables are tender.

6. Meanwhile, cook the quinoa according to package instructions.

7. Remove curry from heat and stir in the chopped cilantro.

8. Serve the chicken and vegetable curry over a bed of the cooked quinoa with lime wedges on the side.

This flavorful curry is loaded with lean protein from the chicken as well as lots of nutritious veggies. The quinoa makes a perfect nutty base to soak up all the delicious coconut curry sauce. You can adjust the heat level by increasing or decreasing the curry powder and cayenne. Delicious and satisfying!

38. Roasted cauliflower and chickpea salad

Ingredients:
- 1 head cauliflower, cut into florets
- 1 (15oz) can chickpeas, drained and rinsed
- 3 tbsp olive oil, divided
- 1 tsp cumin
- 1 tsp paprika
- 1/2 tsp garlic powder
- Salt and pepper to taste
- 1/4 cup dried cranberries or raisins
- 1/4 cup sliced almonds
- 2 cups arugula or spinach
- 1/4 cup crumbled feta cheese

For the Dressing:
- 3 tbsp olive oil
- 2 tbsp lemon juice
- 1 tbsp dijon mustard
- 1 clove garlic, minced
- 1 tbsp honey or maple syrup
- Salt and pepper to taste

Instructions:
1. Preheat oven to 425°F. Line a baking sheet with parchment paper or foil.

2. In a large bowl, toss the cauliflower florets and drained chickpeas with 2 tbsp olive oil, cumin, paprika, garlic powder and a pinch each of salt and pepper.

3. Spread out evenly on the prepared baking sheet. Roast for 20-25 minutes, stirring halfway, until cauliflower is tender and chickpeas are slightly crispy.

4. Meanwhile, make the dressing by whisking together 3 tbsp olive oil, lemon juice, mustard, garlic, honey and salt/pepper to taste.

5. Once vegetables are roasted, transfer to a large bowl and allow to slightly cool for 5 minutes.

6. Add the dried cranberries, sliced almonds, arugula/spinach and feta cheese. Drizzle the salad dressing over top and gently toss everything together to coat. Adjust seasoning with salt, pepper, olive oil or lemon juice if needed.

This hearty salad combines crispy roasted cauliflower and chickpeas with peppery greens, crunchy almonds, sweet cranberries and tangy feta. The lemon honey mustard dressing ties all the flavors together. It's a delicious meatless meal salad that is packed with plant-based protein, fiber and nutrients. Great for lunch or a light dinner.

39. Turkey and vegetable stir-fry with brown rice

Ingredients:
- 1 lb ground turkey
- 2 tbsp sesame oil, divided
- 3 cloves garlic, minced
- 1 tbsp grated ginger
- 1 red bell pepper, sliced
- 1 cup broccoli florets
- 1 cup sliced mushrooms
- 1 cup snap or snow peas
- 3 green onions, sliced
- 2 tbsp low-sodium soy sauce
- 2 tsp rice vinegar
- 1 tsp sesame seeds
- Cooked brown rice, for serving

Instructions:
1. Cook brown rice according to package instructions. Keep warm until ready to serve.

2. Heat 1 tbsp sesame oil in a large skillet or wok over medium-high heat. Add the ground turkey and cook while crumbling with a wooden spoon until browned and cooked through, about 5-7 minutes. Transfer turkey to a plate.

3. Add the remaining 1 tbsp sesame oil to the skillet/wok. Add the garlic and ginger and stir-fry for 30 seconds until fragrant.

4. Add the sliced bell pepper, broccoli, mushrooms and peas. Stir-fry for 3-4 minutes until veggies are crisp-tender.

5. Return the cooked turkey to the skillet/wok along with the green onions.

6. In a small bowl, whisk together the soy sauce, rice vinegar and sesame seeds. Pour over the turkey and veggie mixture and toss everything to combine well.

7. Serve the turkey veggie stir-fry immediately over bowls of warm brown rice. Garnish with extra sesame seeds if desired.

This turkey and veggie stir-fry is a healthy, protein-packed meal loaded with fresh flavors. The lean ground turkey pairs nicely with the crisp-tender veggies for a colorful, nutritious dish. Serving it over brown rice makes it extra satisfying. Feel free to mix up the veggie varieties based on your preference or what you have on hand.

40. Lentil soup with carrots and celery

Ingredients:
- 1 cup dried green or brown lentils, rinsed
- 1 tbsp olive oil
- 1 onion, diced
- 3 carrots, peeled and sliced
- 3 stalks celery, sliced
- 3 cloves garlic, minced
- 1 tsp dried thyme
- 1 bay leaf
- 6 cups vegetable or chicken broth
- 2 cups water
- 1 (14.5 oz) can diced tomatoes
- 1 tsp red wine vinegar
- Salt and pepper to taste
- Chopped parsley for garnish

Instructions:

1. In a large pot or dutch oven, heat the olive oil over medium heat. Add the onions and sauté for 2-3 minutes until translucent.

2. Add the carrots, celery, garlic, thyme and bay leaf. Cook for 3-4 more minutes.

3. Pour in the lentils, broth, water and diced tomatoes with their juices. Bring to a simmer.

4. Reduce heat to medium-low and simmer uncovered for 25-30 minutes, until lentils are very soft and soup has thickened slightly.

5. Remove the bay leaf. Stir in the red wine vinegar and season to taste with salt and pepper.

6. If desired, use an immersion blender to partially blend some of the soup for a creamy texture (or leave it chunky).

7. Ladle soup into bowls and garnish with chopped parsley before serving.

This hearty, protein-packed lentil soup is made extra flavorful from the aromatic veggies like carrots, celery and garlic. It's the perfect comforting soup, especially on chilly days. You can use vegetable or chicken broth based on your preference. Serve it with some crusty bread for dunking. Leftovers make great lunch portions too!

41. Baked trout with roasted vegetables

Ingredients:
- 4 whole trout, cleaned and gutted
- 2 tbsp olive oil, plus more for drizzling
- 1 lemon, thinly sliced
- Salt and pepper
- 1 lb baby potatoes, halved
- 1 lb brussels sprouts, trimmed and halved
- 1 red onion, cut into wedges
- 2 carrots, peeled and sliced
- 2 cloves garlic, minced
- 1 tsp dried thyme
- 2 tbsp butter, melted
- Chopped parsley for garnish

Instructions:
1. Preheat oven to 400°F. Line a baking sheet with parchment paper or foil.

2. Pat the trout fillets dry and brush both sides with olive oil. Season inside and out with salt and pepper. Stuff cavity with lemon slices.

3. In a large bowl, toss together the potatoes, brussels sprouts, onion, carrots, garlic, thyme and 2 tbsp olive oil. Season with salt and pepper.

4. Spread the vegetable mixture out on the prepared baking sheet in an even layer.

5. Place the stuffed trout fillets on top of the vegetables.

6. Drizzle the melted butter over the top of the trout.

7. Roast for 20-25 minutes until the trout is opaque and flakes easily with a fork and the vegetables are tender.

8. Transfer the trout and roasted veggies to a serving platter. Garnish with chopped parsley.

This makes an elegant yet easy one-pan meal. The trout gets deliciously flaky and tender while roasting alongside the medley of roasted potatoes, brussels sprouts, carrots and onions. The lemon stuffed inside infuses everything with a bright, fresh flavor. It's a healthy dinner that feels a little fancy but is so simple to prepare. You can use any firm white fish like trout, branzino or red snapper.

42. Eggplant and zucchini gratin

Ingredients:
- 1 large eggplant, sliced into 1/4 inch rounds
- 2 zucchinis, sliced into 1/4 inch rounds
- 2 tsp salt, divided
- 2 cups marinara or tomato sauce
- 1 cup shredded mozzarella cheese
- 1/2 cup grated parmesan cheese
- 2 eggs, beaten
- 1/2 cup milk or cream
- 1/2 tsp dried basil
- 1/4 tsp garlic powder
- Salt and pepper to taste
- 2 tbsp olive oil
- Chopped parsley for garnish

Instructions:
1. Lay the eggplant and zucchini slices out in a single layer and sprinkle with 1 tsp salt. Let sit for 30 minutes to draw out moisture, then pat dry with paper towels.

2. Preheat oven to 375°F. Grease a 9x13 baking dish with olive oil.

3. Layer 1/3 of the eggplant and zucchini slices in the bottom of the prepared dish, overlapping slightly. Top with 1/3 of the marinara sauce.

4. In a bowl, mix together the eggs, milk, remaining 1 tsp salt, basil, garlic powder, and some pepper.

5. Pour 1/3 of the egg mixture over the veggie layer in the dish. Sprinkle 1/3 of the mozzarella and parmesan over top.

6. Repeat the layering two more times - veggies, sauce, egg mixture, cheeses - ending with the cheeses on top.

7. Bake for 35-40 minutes until hot, bubbly and lightly browned on top. Remove from oven and let stand 5-10 minutes before serving. Garnish with chopped parsley.

This vegetable gratin makes a beautiful, rustic side dish or meatless main course. The salting helps remove excess moisture so the eggplant and zucchini bake up perfectly tender. The layering of sauce, veggies, cheeses, and creamy egg mixture creates amazing flavors in every bite. Serve it alongside some crusty bread to soak up all the delicious juices.

43. Spinach and lentil salad with balsamic vinaigrette

Ingredients:
For the Salad:
- 1 cup dried green or brown lentils, rinsed
- 6 cups fresh baby spinach
- 1 cup cherry tomatoes, halved
- 1/2 English cucumber, diced
- 1/4 red onion, thinly sliced
- 1/4 cup crumbled feta cheese

For the Balsamic Vinaigrette:
- 1/4 cup balsamic vinegar
- 2 tbsp Dijon mustard
- 1 garlic clove, minced
- 1/2 tsp dried oregano
- 1/4 tsp salt
- 1/4 tsp black pepper
- 1/2 cup olive oil

Instructions:
1. Cook the lentils according to package instructions until tender but still firm. Drain any excess water and let cool slightly.

2. Make the vinaigrette by whisking together the balsamic vinegar, mustard, garlic, oregano, salt and pepper in a bowl. Slowly drizzle in the olive oil while whisking continuously until emulsified.

3. In a large bowl, combine the cooked lentils, spinach, cherry tomatoes, cucumber, red onion and feta cheese.

4. Drizzle the balsamic vinaigrette over the salad and toss gently to coat.

5. Let the salad sit for 5-10 minutes to allow the flavors to meld.

6. Give it one more gentle toss and transfer to a serving bowl or plate. Serve immediately.

This hearty spinach and lentil salad makes a wonderfully nutritious vegetarian meal. The lentils provide plant-based protein while the fresh veggies add great crunch and flavor. The tangy balsamic vinaigrette complements everything beautifully. You can enjoy it right away or let it marinate briefly to soften the spinach a bit more. So satisfying and delicious!

44. Quinoa and black bean chili

Ingredients:
- 1 tbsp olive oil
- 1 onion, diced
- 3 cloves garlic, minced
- 2 carrots, peeled and diced
- 2 bell peppers, diced
- 2 tbsp chili powder
- 1 tbsp ground cumin
- 1 tsp dried oregano
- 1/4 tsp cayenne pepper (or more for extra heat)
- 1 (28oz) can diced tomatoes
- 2 (15oz) cans black beans, drained and rinsed
- 4 cups vegetable or chicken broth
- 1 cup quinoa, rinsed
- Salt and pepper to taste
- Toppings: avocado, cheese, sour cream, jalapeños, etc.

Instructions:

1. In a large pot, heat the olive oil over medium-high heat. Add the onions and sauté for 2-3 minutes until translucent.

2. Add the garlic, carrots, and bell peppers. Cook for 4-5 more minutes until vegetables are slightly softened.

3. Stir in the chili powder, cumin, oregano, and cayenne. Cook for 1 minute until fragrant.

4. Add the diced tomatoes, black beans, broth, and quinoa. Season with salt and pepper to taste.

5. Bring the chili to a boil, then reduce heat and let simmer for 20-25 minutes, until quinoa is cooked through and chili has thickened slightly.

6. Adjust seasoning if needed, adding more salt, pepper, chili powder, etc. to your taste preferences.

7. Serve the chili warm topped with desired garnishes like avocado, shredded cheese, sour cream, jalapeños, etc.

This vegetarian quinoa and black bean chili is hearty, nutritious, and full of smoky chili flavor. The quinoa makes it extra protein-packed while the beans add fiber and texture. It's easy to make it vegan by using vegetable broth. You can also cook up some ground turkey or beef to add into it for extra protein if desired. The toppings make it extra delicious!

45. Grilled chicken Caesar salad with romaine lettuce

Ingredients:
- 2 boneless, skinless chicken breasts
- 2 tbsp olive oil
- 1 tsp dried oregano
- Salt and pepper
- 1 large head romaine lettuce, chopped
- 1 cup croutons
- 1/2 cup grated parmesan cheese, plus more for serving
- ***Caesar Dressing:***
- 1 egg yolk
- 2 anchovy fillets, minced (optional)
- 2 garlic cloves, minced
- 2 tbsp lemon juice
- 1 tsp Dijon mustard
- 1/2 cup olive oil
- 2 tbsp grated parmesan
- Salt and pepper to taste

Instructions:
1. Rub the chicken breasts with 1 tbsp of the olive oil and season with oregano, salt and pepper.

2. Grill the chicken over medium-high heat for 5-7 minutes per side until cooked through. Let rest 5 minutes before slicing.

3. Make the Caesar dressing by whisking together the egg yolk, anchovy fillets (if using), garlic, lemon juice and mustard. Then slowly drizzle in the 1/2 cup olive oil while whisking continuously until emulsified. Whisk in the 2 tbsp parmesan and season with salt and pepper.

4. In a large bowl, toss the chopped romaine lettuce with the croutons, sliced grilled chicken and 1/2 cup parmesan cheese.

5. Pour the desired amount of Caesar dressing over the salad and toss to coat everything evenly. Transfer to a serving bowl or plate and top with extra parmesan cheese.

The grilled chicken adds wonderful smoky flavor while the crisp romaine contrasts nicely with the rich, creamy Caesar dressing. Crunchy croutons and shaved parmesan make this salad ultra satisfying. It's a protein-packed entree salad perfect for lunch or dinner. You can also grill some slices of bread rubbed with garlic to serve alongside.

46. Stir-fried tofu with broccoli and bell peppers

Ingredients:
- 14 oz extra-firm tofu, drained and cubed
- 2 tbsp soy sauce or tamari, plus more for drizzling
- 2 tbsp rice vinegar
- 1 tbsp sesame oil
- 2 tsp cornstarch
- 3 tbsp vegetable or peanut oil, divided
- 1 red bell pepper, sliced
- 1 yellow bell pepper, sliced
- 4 cups broccoli florets
- 3 cloves garlic, minced
- 1 tbsp freshly grated ginger
- 2 green onions, sliced
- Cooked rice or quinoa, for serving

Instructions:
1. In a shallow bowl, gently toss the cubed tofu with 2 tbsp soy sauce, rice vinegar, sesame oil and cornstarch until coated. Let marinate for 10 minutes.

2. Heat 2 tbsp of the vegetable oil in a large skillet or wok over high heat. Add the marinated tofu and fry undisturbed for 2-3 minutes to get a crispy exterior.

3. Flip and fry the other side for 2 more minutes. Transfer tofu to a plate.

4. Add the remaining 1 tbsp oil to the skillet/wok, along with the sliced bell peppers and broccoli florets. Stir-fry for 3-4 minutes until lightly charred in spots.

5. Add the garlic, ginger and green onions. Stir-fry for 1 minute until fragrant.

6. Return the fried tofu to the skillet/wok and toss everything together.

7. Remove from heat and drizzle over a bit more soy sauce to taste, if desired.

8. Serve immediately over steamed rice or quinoa.

This veggie-packed stir-fry features crispy baked tofu and fresh broccoli and bell peppers cooked in an aromatic garlic-ginger sauce. It's a flavorful, protein-rich vegetarian/vegan dish. The marinade gives the tofu the most delicious texture and allows it to really soak up all the flavors of the stir-fry. Adjust spice levels by adding crushed chiles if desired.

47. Kale and avocado salad with grilled shrimp

Ingredients:
- 1 bunch kale, stems removed and leaves chopped
- 1 avocado, diced
- 1 pint grape tomatoes, halved
- 1/4 red onion, thinly sliced
- 1 lb shrimp, peeled and deveined
- 2 tbsp olive oil
- 2 tsp cajun or blackening seasoning
- 1 lemon, cut into wedges

For the Dressing:
- 1/4 cup olive oil
- 2 tbsp red wine vinegar
- 1 tsp dijon mustard
- 2 tsp honey
- 1 clove garlic, minced
- Salt and pepper to taste

Instructions:
1. Make the dressing by whisking together the 1/4 cup olive oil, vinegar, mustard, honey, garlic, and salt and pepper to taste. Set aside.

2. In a large bowl, toss together the chopped kale, diced avocado, grape tomatoes, and sliced red onion.

3. Toss the shrimp with the 2 tbsp olive oil and cajun/blackening seasoning until evenly coated.

4. Heat a grill pan or outdoor grill to medium-high heat. Grill the shrimp for 2-3 minutes per side until opaque and cooked through.

5. Transfer the grilled shrimp to the salad bowl with the kale and vegetables.

6. Drizzle the desired amount of dressing over top and gently toss to coat everything evenly.

7. Squeeze fresh lemon juice from the wedges over the salad.

8. Serve the kale and avocado salad with the grilled shrimp immediately, while the shrimp is still warm.

This salad is loaded with fresh, vibrant flavors and makes a wonderful light meal. The slight bitterness of the kale is balanced by the creamy avocado and sweet dressing. The spicy grilled shrimp adds a protein boost and delicious charred flavor. You can make it heartier by adding quinoa or serve it with crusty bread on the side.

48. Baked cod with lemon and herbs

Ingredients:
- 1 1/4 lbs cod fillets
- 2 tbsp olive oil
- 1 lemon, thinly sliced
- 3 cloves garlic, minced
- 1 tsp dried oregano
- 1 tsp dried thyme
- 1/4 cup dry white wine or broth
- Salt and pepper to taste
- 2 tbsp chopped fresh parsley
- Lemon wedges for serving

Instructions:
1. Preheat oven to 400°F. Line a baking sheet with parchment paper or foil.

2. Pat the cod fillets dry and place them on the prepared baking sheet. Brush both sides of the fish with 1 tbsp of the olive oil and season with salt and pepper.

3. In a small bowl, combine the minced garlic, dried oregano, dried thyme and remaining 1 tbsp olive oil.

4. Spread the garlic-herb mixture over the top of the cod fillets.

5. Arrange the lemon slices in a single layer over and around the cod.

6. Pour the white wine or broth into the baking sheet around the fish.

7. Transfer to the oven and bake for 12-15 minutes, until the fish is opaque and flakes easily with a fork.

8. Remove from oven and garnish the baked cod with chopped fresh parsley.

9. Serve immediately with extra lemon wedges for squeezing over top.

This baked cod has such bright, fresh flavors from the garlic, herbs, lemon and white wine. Baking it in the oven keeps the fish tender and flaky on the inside with a light crisp on top. The lemon slices infuse incredible citrusy aroma and taste. It's a healthy, easy meal that feels a little fancy but comes together in under 30 minutes. Serve it over rice or pasta, or with a side of roasted veggies.

49. Moroccan chickpea stew

Ingredients:
- 2 tablespoons olive oil
- 1 large onion, diced
- 4 cloves garlic, minced
- 1 tablespoon ground cumin
- 1 teaspoon ground coriander
- 1 teaspoon ground cinnamon
- 1/4 teaspoon cayenne pepper (or more to taste)
- 1 (15 oz) can diced tomatoes
- 4 cups vegetable or chicken broth
- 2 (15 oz) cans chickpeas, drained and rinsed
- 1 sweet potato, peeled and diced
- 1 cup dried apricots, quartered
- 2 tablespoons lemon juice
- Salt and pepper to taste
- Chopped parsley for garnish

Instructions:
1. In a large pot or dutch oven, heat the olive oil over medium heat. Add the onion and sauté for 5 minutes until translucent.

2. Add the garlic, cumin, coriander, cinnamon and cayenne. Cook for 1 minute until fragrant.

3. Pour in the diced tomatoes and broth. Add the chickpeas, sweet potato, and apricots.

4. Season with salt and pepper to taste.

5. Bring to a boil, then reduce heat and simmer for 20-25 minutes until sweet potatoes are tender.

6. Remove from heat and stir in the lemon juice. Garnish with chopped parsley. Serve over couscous or with crusty bread if desired.

This hearty stew has a wonderful blend of Moroccan spices along with the sweetness from the apricots and sweet potatoes. It makes a flavorful vegetarian or vegan meal. Enjoy!

50. Spaghetti squash primavera with grilled chicken

Ingredients:
- 1 medium spaghetti squash
- 2 tablespoons olive oil, divided
- 1 lb boneless, skinless chicken breasts
- 1 teaspoon Italian seasoning
- Salt and pepper to taste
- 2 cups broccoli florets
- 1 cup sliced zucchini
- 1 cup sliced yellow squash
- 1 red bell pepper, julienned
- 3 cloves garlic, minced
- 1 cup halved cherry tomatoes
- 1/4 cup vegetable or chicken broth
- 2 tablespoons lemon juice
- 1/4 cup grated parmesan cheese
- 2 tablespoons chopped fresh basil

Instructions:

1. Preheat oven to 400°F. Cut spaghetti squash in half lengthwise and scoop out seeds. Brush the insides with 1 tbsp olive oil and season with salt and pepper. Place cut-side down on a baking sheet and roast for 40-50 minutes until tender. Allow to cool slightly.

2. Brush the chicken breasts with the remaining 1 tbsp olive oil and season with Italian seasoning, salt and pepper. Grill over medium-high heat for 5-7 minutes per side until cooked through. Let rest 5 minutes then slice into strips.

3. Use a fork to scrape the flesh of the spaghetti squash into spaghetti-like strands and transfer to a large bowl.

4. Bring a pot of salted water to a boil and cook the broccoli florets for 2-3 minutes until crisp-tender. Drain and add to the spaghetti squash.

5. In a large skillet, sauté the zucchini, yellow squash, bell pepper and garlic for 3-4 minutes over medium-high heat until tender-crisp.

6. Add the veggies to the spaghetti squash along with the sliced chicken, cherry tomatoes, broth and lemon juice. Toss to combine.

7. Transfer to a serving dish and top with grated parmesan and fresh basil before serving.

This primavera style dish is a lighter, low-carb way to enjoy pasta using healthy spaghetti squash as the base. The grilled chicken adds protein and the fresh veggies make it a complete, flavorful meal. Enjoy!

51. Grilled salmon with a quinoa and kale salad

Ingredients:
For the Salmon:
- 4 (6oz) salmon fillets
- 2 tbsp olive oil
- 1 tsp lemon pepper seasoning
- Salt and pepper to taste

For the Quinoa Salad:
- 1 cup quinoa, rinsed
- 2 cups vegetable or chicken broth
- 4 cups packed kale, stems removed and chopped
- 1 cup halved cherry tomatoes
- 1/2 cup sliced cucumber
- 1/4 cup crumbled feta cheese
- 2 tbsp olive oil
- 2 tbsp lemon juice
- 1 clove garlic, minced
- Salt and pepper to taste

Instructions:
1. Rinse the quinoa in a mesh strainer. In a saucepan, combine the quinoa and broth. Bring to a boil, then reduce heat to low, cover and simmer for 15-20 minutes until liquid is absorbed. Fluff with a fork and set aside to cool slightly.

2. In a large bowl, combine the cooked quinoa, chopped kale, tomatoes, cucumber and feta.

3. In a small bowl, whisk together the olive oil, lemon juice, garlic and season with salt and pepper. Pour the dressing over the quinoa salad and toss to coat.

4. Brush the salmon fillets with olive oil and season with lemon pepper, salt and pepper.

5. Grill the salmon over medium-high heat for 4-5 minutes per side until cooked through and flaky.

6. To serve, place a salmon fillet over a bed of the quinoa and kale salad.

The grilled salmon pairs beautifully with the fresh quinoa salad loaded with nutrient-dense kale, tomatoes, cucumber and feta cheese. The lemon dressing helps brighten all the flavors. This makes a healthy, protein-packed meal that is gluten-free and full of superfoods like salmon and kale. Enjoy!

52. Sweet potato and black bean enchiladas

Ingredients:
- Salt and pepper to taste
- 2 (15 oz) cans black beans, drained and rinsed
- 1 cup frozen corn
- 8-10 tortillas (corn or flour)
- 2 cups enchilada sauce
- 2 cups shredded Mexican cheese blend
- Diced avocado, chopped cilantro, lime wedges for serving
- 3 medium sweet potatoes, peeled and diced into 1/2-inch cubes
- 2 tablespoons olive oil, divided
- 1 red onion, diced
- 3 cloves garlic, minced
- 2 teaspoons ground cumin
- 1 teaspoon chili powder
- 1/2 teaspoon smoked paprika

Instructions:

1. Preheat oven to 400°F. Toss the diced sweet potatoes with 1 tbsp olive oil and spread on a baking sheet. Roast for 20-25 minutes until tender.

2. In a skillet, heat the remaining 1 tbsp olive oil over medium heat. Sauté the onion until soft, about 5 minutes.

3. Add the garlic and spices (cumin, chili powder, paprika) and cook for 1 minute until fragrant.

4. Stir in the black beans, roasted sweet potatoes, and frozen corn. Season with salt and pepper to taste.

5. Warm the tortillas according to package instructions to make them pliable for rolling.

6. Spread 1/2 cup enchilada sauce in the bottom of a 9x13 baking dish.

7. Place about 1/3 cup of the sweet potato black bean filling into each tortilla, roll up tightly and place seam-side down in the baking dish.

8. Pour the remaining enchilada sauce over the top and sprinkle with the shredded cheese. Bake for 20 minutes until heated through and the cheese is melted. Serve warm, topped with diced avocado, chopped cilantro and lime wedges if desired.

These enchiladas are packed with fiber and plant-based protein from the black beans and sweet potatoes. The Mexican spices add tons of flavor. They make a delicious vegetarian meal! You can also add shredded chicken to make them non-vegetarian if desired.

53. Roasted chicken breast with steamed spinach

Ingredients:
- 4 boneless, skinless chicken breasts
- 2 tablespoons olive oil
- 1 teaspoon paprika
- 1 teaspoon garlic powder
- Salt and pepper to taste

- 1 lb fresh spinach
- 1 tablespoon olive oil
- 2 cloves garlic, minced
- 1 tablespoon lemon juice
- Salt and pepper to taste

Instructions:
For the Roasted Chicken:
1. Preheat oven to 400°F (200°C).

2. Pound the chicken breasts lightly so they are of even thickness. This will help them cook evenly.

3. In a small bowl, mix together olive oil, paprika, garlic powder, and salt and pepper.

4. Rub the seasoning mixture all over the chicken breasts.

5. Place the chicken on a baking sheet lined with foil or parchment paper.

6. Roast for 20-25 minutes until chicken is cooked through (165°F internal temp). Let rest 5 minutes before serving.

For the Steamed Spinach:
1. In a large pot or dutch oven, bring 1 inch of water to a simmer over medium heat.

2. Add the spinach and cover with a lid. Steam for 2-3 minutes until wilted.

3. Drain the spinach well and transfer to a bowl.

4. Toss the spinach with olive oil, minced garlic, lemon juice and salt and pepper to taste.

To Serve: Slice the roasted chicken breasts and serve alongside the steamed garlic-lemon spinach.

This makes a simple, lean, and nutritious meal. The roasted chicken is moist and flavorful thanks to the paprika seasoning. The garlicky spinach with a pop of lemon adds freshness and vital nutrients. It's an easy but satisfying dinner!

54. Chickpea and spinach stew

Ingredients:
- 2 tablespoons olive oil
- 1 large onion, diced
- 4 cloves garlic, minced
- 1 tablespoon ground cumin
- 1 teaspoon smoked paprika
- 1/4 teaspoon cayenne pepper (optional)
- 2 (15oz) cans chickpeas, drained and rinsed
- 1 (15oz) can diced tomatoes
- 4 cups vegetable or chicken broth
- 1 bunch spinach, washed and roughly chopped
- Salt and pepper to taste
- Juice of 1/2 a lemon
- Chopped parsley for garnish
- Crusty bread for serving

Instructions:

1. In a large pot or dutch oven, heat the olive oil over medium heat. Add the diced onion and cook for 5 minutes until translucent.

2. Add the garlic, cumin, smoked paprika and cayenne (if using). Cook for 1 minute until fragrant.

3. Pour in the chickpeas, diced tomatoes and broth. Season with salt and pepper to taste.

4. Bring the stew to a boil, then reduce heat and let simmer for 15 minutes, stirring occasionally.

5. Add the chopped spinach and let wilt for 2-3 minutes, stirring it into the stew as it wilts down.

6. Remove stew from heat and stir in the fresh lemon juice. Taste and adjust seasoning as needed. Ladle into bowls and garnish with chopped parsley. Serve with crusty bread on the side.

This vegetarian stew is loaded with plant-based protein from the chickpeas along with fiber, vitamins and minerals from the spinach, tomatoes and aromatics. The smoky paprika and cumin add warmth and depth of flavor. It makes a comforting, healthy meal that packs well for lunches too. You can also add cooked chicken or sausage to make it non-vegetarian if desired. Enjoy!

55. Grilled mackerel with a mixed green salad

Ingredients:
- 4 whole mackerel fillets
- 2 tablespoons olive oil
- 1 teaspoon lemon pepper seasoning
- Salt and pepper to taste

For the Salad:
- 5 oz mixed greens
- 1 cup cherry tomatoes, halved
- 1/2 English cucumber, sliced
- 1/4 red onion, thinly sliced
- 1/4 cup crumbled feta cheese
- 2 tablespoons olive oil
- 1 tablespoon red wine vinegar
- 1 teaspoon Dijon mustard
- 1 clove garlic, minced
- Salt and pepper to taste

Instructions:
For the Mackerel:
1. Rinse the mackerel fillets and pat them dry. Brush both sides with olive oil and season with lemon pepper, salt and pepper. Preheat grill or grill pan to medium-high heat.

2. Grill the mackerel for 3-4 minutes per side until fish is opaque and flakes easily with a fork. Transfer grilled mackerel to a plate and cover loosely with foil to keep warm.

For the Salad:
1. In a large bowl, combine the mixed greens, cherry tomatoes, cucumber, red onion and feta.

2. In a small bowl, whisk together the olive oil, red wine vinegar, Dijon mustard, garlic and season with salt and pepper. Drizzle the vinaigrette over the salad and toss gently to coat.

Divide the mixed green salad between plates and top with the grilled mackerel fillets.

Grilling mackerel gives it a wonderful smoky flavor and crispy skin. The salad with fresh veggies, feta and tangy vinaigrette makes the perfect light and healthy accompaniment. Mackerel is an excellent source of heart-healthy omega-3 fatty acids. This meal is gluten-free, low-carb and loaded with nutrients. Enjoy!

56. Tofu and vegetable curry with brown rice

Ingredients:
- 1 block (14oz) extra-firm tofu, pressed and cubed
- 2 tablespoons oil (vegetable, coconut or olive oil)
- 1 onion, diced
- 3 cloves garlic, minced
- 1 tbsp grated fresh ginger
- 2 tbsp curry powder
- 1 tsp garam masala
- 1 tsp ground cumin
- 1 (15oz) can crushed tomatoes
- 1 (15oz) can full-fat coconut milk
- 1 cup vegetable broth or water
- 1 bell pepper, diced
- 2 cups diced vegetables (potato, carrots, cauliflower etc.)
- Juice of 1/2 lemon
- Salt and pepper to taste
- Chopped cilantro for garnish
- Cooked brown rice, for serving

Instructions:

1. Press the tofu for 20-30 minutes to remove excess moisture. Then cut into 1-inch cubes.

2. In a large pot or dutch oven, heat the oil over medium-high heat. Add the cubed tofu and fry for 2-3 minutes until lightly browned on all sides. Remove tofu from pot and set aside.

3. In the same pot, sauté the onion for 2-3 minutes until translucent. Add the garlic and grated ginger and cook for 1 minute until fragrant.

4. Stir in the curry powder, garam masala, cumin and crushed tomatoes. Cook for 2 minutes, stirring frequently.

5. Pour in the coconut milk and vegetable broth. Add the diced bell pepper and other vegetables.

6. Return the tofu to the pot and stir to combine everything. Season with salt and pepper to taste.

7. Bring to a simmer, then reduce heat to low, cover and simmer for 15-20 minutes until vegetables are tender.

8. Remove from heat and stir in the lemon juice. Serve the curry over brown rice and garnish with chopped fresh cilantro.

This vegetable-packed curry is full of aromatic spices like curry, cumin and garam masala. The tofu adds plant-based protein while the coconut milk creates a rich, creamy sauce. Serve it over nutty brown rice for a satisfying, flavorful vegetarian/vegan meal. Adjust spice level to taste. Enjoy!

57. Lentil and quinoa salad with fresh herbs

Ingredients:
- 1 cup dried green or brown lentils, rinsed and picked over
- 1/2 cup quinoa, rinsed
- 1 cup cherry tomatoes, halved
- 1 cucumber, diced
- 1/2 red onion, finely diced
- 1/2 cup chopped fresh parsley
- 1/4 cup chopped fresh mint
- 2 tablespoons chopped fresh dill
- Juice of 1 lemon
- 3 tablespoons olive oil
- 2 cloves garlic, minced
- 1 teaspoon Dijon mustard
- Salt and pepper to taste

Instructions:

1. In a saucepan, cover the lentils with 2 cups of water or vegetable broth. Bring to a boil, then reduce heat and simmer for 15-20 minutes until lentils are tender but still hold their shape. Drain any excess liquid.

2. While the lentils cook, rinse the quinoa thoroughly. In another saucepan, combine the quinoa with 1 cup of water or broth and a pinch of salt. Bring to a boil, then reduce heat to low, cover and simmer for 15 minutes. Remove from heat and let sit covered for 5 more minutes. Fluff with a fork.

3. Transfer the cooked lentils and quinoa to a large bowl and allow to cool slightly.

4. Add the cherry tomatoes, cucumber, red onion, parsley, mint and dill. Toss to combine.

5. Make the dressing by whisking together the lemon juice, olive oil, minced garlic, Dijon and salt/pepper to taste.

6. Pour the dressing over the lentil-quinoa salad and toss gently to coat. Let the salad marinate for at least 30 minutes to allow the flavors to meld. Taste and adjust seasoning as needed before serving. Enjoy!

This lentil and quinoa salad is a protein-packed vegetarian delight. The fresh herbs add a vibrant flavor along with the tangy lemon dressing. It's a great make-ahead dish that keeps well for lunches or potlucks. The fiber and nutrients make it a healthy and satisfying meal on its own or a tasty side salad.

58. Baked zucchini boats stuffed with ground turkey

Ingredients:
- 4 medium zucchinis
- 1 tbsp olive oil
- 1 lb ground turkey
- 1/2 onion, diced
- 3 cloves garlic, minced
- 1 cup marinara sauce
- 1/2 cup cooked quinoa or rice
- 1/2 cup shredded mozzarella cheese
- 1/4 cup grated parmesan cheese
- 2 tbsp chopped fresh basil
- Salt and pepper to taste

Instructions:

1. Preheat oven to 400°F (200°C). Cut the zucchinis in half lengthwise and use a spoon to hollow out the center, leaving about 1/2 inch thickness on the sides. Place the zucchini halves on a baking sheet.

2. In a skillet, heat the olive oil over medium-high heat. Add the ground turkey and onions. Cook while crumbling the turkey until no longer pink, about 5-7 minutes.

3. Add the garlic and cook for 1 minute until fragrant.

4. Stir in the marinara sauce and cooked quinoa or rice. Season with salt and pepper to taste.

5. Stuff each hollowed zucchini half with the ground turkey marinara mixture.

6. Top each stuffed zucchini boat with shredded mozzarella and grated parmesan cheese.

7. Bake for 20-25 minutes until the zucchini is fork tender and the cheese is melted and lightly browned.

8. Remove from oven and sprinkle with chopped fresh basil before serving.

These zucchini boats are a delicious way to enjoy ground turkey with Italian flavors. The zucchini provides a low-carb base while the filling is protein-packed and flavorful from the marinara and cheeses. You can easily make it vegetarian by stuffing with marinara and veggies instead of turkey. Serve these as a tasty main dish or a fun appetizer!

59. Cauliflower and chickpea curry

Ingredients:
- 1 head cauliflower, cut into florets
- 1 (15oz) can chickpeas, drained and rinsed
- 2 tablespoons olive oil
- 1 onion, diced
- 3 cloves garlic, minced
- 1 tablespoon grated fresh ginger
- 1 tablespoon curry powder
- 1 teaspoon garam masala
- 1 teaspoon ground cumin
- 1 teaspoon ground coriander
- 1 (15oz) can crushed tomatoes
- 1 cup vegetable or chicken broth
- 1 (15oz) can full-fat coconut milk
- 1 cup frozen peas
- Salt and pepper to taste
- Chopped cilantro for garnish
- Cooked basmati rice, for serving

Instructions:

1. In a large pot or dutch oven, heat the olive oil over medium-high heat. Add the diced onion and cook for 2-3 minutes until translucent.

2. Add the garlic, ginger, curry powder, garam masala, cumin and coriander. Cook for 1-2 minutes until fragrant.

3. Pour in the crushed tomatoes and broth. Stir to combine.

4. Add the cauliflower florets and chickpeas. Season with salt and pepper to taste.

5. Bring the curry to a simmer, then reduce heat to medium-low. Cover and simmer for 15 minutes, stirring occasionally.

6. Pour in the coconut milk and frozen peas. Simmer for 5 more minutes.

7. Taste and adjust seasoning as needed, adding more salt, pepper or spices to your taste preferences.

8. Serve the curry over basmati rice, garnished with chopped fresh cilantro.

This flavorful vegetarian curry is loaded with cauliflower, protein-packed chickpeas, aromatic spices and creamy coconut milk. It makes a hearty, satisfying and nutritious meat-free meal. The peas add a pop of color and freshness. You can easily make it vegan by using vegetable broth. Adjust the heat level by adjusting the amount of curry powder. Delicious and comforting!

60. Salmon and avocado sushi rolls

Ingredients:
- 4 sheets sushi nori (seaweed sheets)
- 1 cup sushi rice, cooked per package instructions
- 1 ripe avocado, sliced
- 4 oz smoked salmon, sliced into strips
- 2 tablespoons rice vinegar
- 1 tablespoon sesame seeds
- Soy sauce, wasabi and pickled ginger for serving

Instructions:
1. Once the sushi rice is cooked and still warm, transfer it to a bowl and mix in the rice vinegar until well combined. Allow to cool slightly.

2. Place a sushi mat or thin towel on a flat surface. Have a small bowl of cold water nearby to dip your fingers in to help spread the rice.

3. Place one nori sheet shiny side down on the mat. Dip your fingers in water and spread 1/4 of the sushi rice in an even thin layer over the nori, leaving a 1-inch border at the top.

4. In the center of the rice, lay a few strips of smoked salmon and some sliced avocado in a line horizontally.

5. Using the mat, carefully roll up the nori tightly starting from the bottom, using the mat to squeeze the roll firmly together.

6. Once rolled, dab a little water on the end border to seal the roll closed.

7. Sprinkle sesame seeds over the roll and let sit seam side down.

8. Repeat with remaining nori, rice, salmon and avocado to make 4 rolls total.

9. Using a very sharp knife, slice each roll into 6-8 pieces.

10. Serve the sushi rolls immediately with soy sauce, wasabi and pickled ginger for dipping.

These fresh salmon and avocado rolls make a delicious handheld sushi! The smoked salmon provides richness while the avocado adds creaminess. You can add other fillings like cucumber or mango if desired. Learning to roll sushi at home is a fun skill to master. Just be sure to have all your fillings prepped before assembling the rolls.

61. Quinoa and vegetable stuffed mushrooms

Ingredients:
- 2 cloves garlic, minced
- 1 cup finely chopped spinach or kale
- 1/4 cup grated parmesan cheese
- 2 tbsp breadcrumbs
- 2 tbsp chopped fresh parsley
- 1 tsp dried thyme
- Salt and pepper to taste
- 16-20 large mushrooms (cremini or portobello), stems removed and chopped
- 2 tbsp olive oil, divided
- 1 cup cooked quinoa
- 1/2 cup finely chopped bell pepper
- 1/2 cup finely chopped onion

Instructions:

1. Preheat oven to 375°F (190°C). Lightly grease a baking sheet or dish.

2. Clean the mushroom caps and remove the stems. Finely chop the stems.

3. In a skillet, heat 1 tbsp of the olive oil over medium heat. Sauté the chopped mushroom stems, bell pepper, and onion until softened, about 5 minutes.

4. Add the garlic and sauté for 1 minute until fragrant. Then add the chopped spinach/kale and cook for 2 more minutes until wilted.

5. Remove the veggie mixture from heat and stir in the cooked quinoa, parmesan, breadcrumbs, parsley, thyme and salt and pepper to taste.

6. Brush the mushroom caps with the remaining 1 tbsp olive oil on both sides.

7. Mound the quinoa stuffing into each mushroom cap cavity, pressing gently to make it compact.

8. Arrange the stuffed mushrooms on the prepared baking sheet/dish.

9. Bake for 18-20 minutes until mushrooms are tender and stuffing is lightly browned on top. Serve the stuffed mushrooms warm, garnished with extra parsley if desired.

These vegetable stuffed mushrooms are nutrient-dense, protein-packed and absolutely delicious! The quinoa makes a fantastic filling with all the chopped veggies, parmesan and herbs. They make a tasty vegetarian appetizer or you can serve several stuffed mushrooms as a light main dish. Enjoy!

62. Grilled tuna steak with roasted vegetables

Ingredients:
- 4 tuna steaks (6-8 oz each)
- 2 tbsp olive oil, plus more for vegetables
- 1 tbsp lemon juice
- 2 cloves garlic, minced
- 1 tsp dried oregano
- Salt and pepper to taste
- 1 zucchini, halved lengthwise and sliced 1/2-inch thick
- 1 red bell pepper, seeded and cut into 1-inch pieces
- 1 red onion, cut into wedges
- 1 lb baby potatoes, halved
- 2 tbsp balsamic vinegar

Instructions:

For the Tuna:

1. Rinse the tuna steaks and pat them dry. Place in a shallow dish.

2. In a small bowl, whisk together 2 tbsp olive oil, lemon juice, garlic, oregano, and salt and pepper.

3. Pour the marinade over the tuna steaks and turn to coat both sides. Cover and marinate for 20-30 minutes at room temperature.

4. Preheat grill or grill pan to high heat and brush grates with oil.

5. Grill the tuna for 2-3 minutes per side for rare, or longer if you prefer more doneness.

6. Transfer tuna to a plate, cover loosely with foil and let rest 5 minutes before serving.

For the Roasted Veggies:

1. Preheat oven to 400°F (200°C). Line a baking sheet with foil or parchment paper.

2. In a large bowl, toss the zucchini, bell pepper, onion and potatoes with 2-3 tbsp olive oil and salt/pepper to taste.

3. Spread the vegetables out in an even layer on the prepared baking sheet.

4. Roast for 20 minutes, then toss and roast 10 more minutes until tender and browning.

5. Transfer roasted veggies to a bowl and toss with the balsamic vinegar.

Slice the grilled tuna steaks and serve alongside the roasted balsamic vegetables. The freshness of the tuna pairs beautifully with the sweet caramelized roasted veggies! Garnish with extra lemon if desired. Enjoy!

63. Chickpea and vegetable stir-fry with brown rice

Ingredients:
- 2 carrots, julienned
- 3 cloves garlic, minced
- 1 tbsp grated fresh ginger
- 2 tbsp soy sauce or tamari
- 1 tbsp rice vinegar
- 1 tsp sesame seeds (optional)
- 2 green onions, sliced (optional)
- 1 cup dry brown rice, cooked per package instructions
- 1 (15oz) can chickpeas, drained and rinsed
- 2 tbsp sesame oil or vegetable oil
- 1 red bell pepper, sliced
- 1 cup broccoli florets
- 1 cup sliced mushrooms
- 1 cup snap or snow peas

Instructions:

1. Cook the brown rice per package instructions. Keep covered to stay warm after cooking.

2. Heat the sesame or vegetable oil in a large skillet or wok over high heat.

3. Add the sliced bell pepper, broccoli, mushrooms, peas, carrots and chickpeas. Stir-fry for 3-4 minutes until veggies are crisp tender.

4. Push the veggies to the sides and make a well in the center of the pan. Allow to heat up, then add the garlic and grated ginger. Cook for 30 seconds until fragrant.

5. Drizzle in the soy sauce and rice vinegar. Toss everything together and continue to stir-fry for 1-2 minutes more.

6. Remove stir-fry from heat. Taste and adjust any seasoning as needed, adding more soy sauce if desired.

7. Serve the chickpea and veggie stir-fry over the cooked brown rice. Garnish with sesame seeds and sliced green onions if desired.

This veggie-packed stir-fry is a nutritious and protein-rich meatless meal thanks to the addition of chickpeas. The fresh ginger, garlic and soy sauce give it so much flavor. Using brown rice makes it a fiber-filled, hearty dish. You can easily substitute other veggies you have on hand like snap or snow peas, bok choy, cabbage etc. It's a fantastic way to use up leftover cooked rice and frozen veggie medleys too. Enjoy!

64. Turkey and vegetable soup

Ingredients:
- 2 tablespoons olive oil
- 1 onion, chopped
- 2 carrots, chopped
- 2 celery stalks, chopped
- 3 cloves garlic, minced
- 1 teaspoon dried thyme
- 1 teaspoon dried oregano
- 1 teaspoon dried rosemary
- Salt and pepper to taste
- 8 cups turkey or chicken broth
- 2 cups cooked turkey, shredded or diced
- 1 can (14 oz) diced tomatoes
- 1 cup green beans, trimmed and cut into bite-sized pieces
- 1 cup corn kernels (fresh, canned, or frozen)
- 1 cup peas (fresh, canned, or frozen)
- 2 cups spinach leaves, chopped
- Fresh parsley, chopped (for garnish)
- Grated Parmesan cheese (optional, for garnish)

Instructions:

1. Heat olive oil in a large pot over medium heat. Add chopped onions, carrots, and celery. Cook until vegetables are softened, about 5-7 minutes.

2. Add minced garlic, dried thyme, oregano, and rosemary to the pot. Stir and cook for another minute until fragrant.

3. Season with salt and pepper to taste.

4. Pour in turkey or chicken broth and bring the mixture to a boil.

5. Once boiling, reduce heat to low and add cooked turkey, diced tomatoes (with their juices), green beans, corn, and peas to the pot. Simmer for about 15-20 minutes until vegetables are tender.

6. Stir in chopped spinach leaves and cook for an additional 2-3 minutes until wilted.

7. Taste and adjust seasoning if needed.

8. Ladle the soup into bowls and garnish with chopped parsley and grated Parmesan cheese if desired. Serve hot and enjoy!

This soup is perfect for using up leftover turkey from Thanksgiving or any other occasion, and it's packed with nutritious vegetables. Feel free to customize the recipe by adding your favorite herbs or swapping out vegetables based on what you have on hand. Enjoy!

65. Baked haddock with a side of green beans

Ingredients:
- 4 haddock fillets (about 6 oz each)
- 2 tablespoons olive oil
- 2 cloves garlic, minced
- 1 teaspoon paprika
- 1 teaspoon dried thyme
- 1 teaspoon dried parsley
- Salt and pepper to taste
- 1 lemon, sliced
- 1 lb fresh green beans, trimmed
- 2 tablespoons grated Parmesan cheese (optional, for garnish)
- Fresh parsley, chopped (for garnish)

Instructions:

1. Preheat your oven to 375°F (190°C). Line a baking sheet with parchment paper or lightly grease it with olive oil.

2. Place the haddock fillets on the prepared baking sheet, leaving space between each fillet.

3. In a small bowl, mix together olive oil, minced garlic, paprika, dried thyme, dried parsley, salt, and pepper.

4. Brush the olive oil mixture evenly over the haddock fillets.

5. Arrange lemon slices on top of each fillet.

6. Place the baking sheet in the preheated oven and bake for about 15-20 minutes, or until the fish is cooked through and flakes easily with a fork.

7. While the haddock is baking, prepare the green beans. Bring a pot of salted water to a boil. Add the trimmed green beans and cook for about 3-4 minutes, or until they are crisp-tender. Drain the beans and set aside.

8. Once the haddock is done baking, remove it from the oven and let it rest for a few minutes.

9. Serve the baked haddock hot, garnished with grated Parmesan cheese (if using) and chopped parsley, alongside the cooked green beans. Enjoy your flavorful and nutritious meal!

This recipe provides a simple and delicious way to enjoy haddock, and the side of green beans adds freshness and crunch to the dish. Feel free to adjust the seasonings or add your favorite herbs and spices to suit your taste preferences.

66. Eggplant and chickpea stew

Ingredients:
- 2 medium eggplants, diced
- 1 can (15 oz) chickpeas,
drained and rinsed
- 1 onion, diced
- 3 cloves garlic, minced
- 1 can (14 oz) diced tomatoes
- 2 tablespoons tomato paste
- 1 teaspoon ground cumin
- 1 teaspoon ground coriander
- 1 teaspoon smoked paprika
- 1/2 teaspoon chili powder (adjust to taste)
- Salt and pepper to taste
- 2 cups vegetable broth
- 2 tablespoons olive oil
- Fresh parsley or cilantro, chopped (for garnish)

Instructions:

1. Heat olive oil in a large pot or Dutch oven over medium heat. Add diced onion and minced garlic. Cook until onion is soft and translucent, about 5 minutes.

2. Add diced eggplant to the pot. Cook, stirring occasionally, until the eggplant starts to soften, about 5-7 minutes.

3. Stir in ground cumin, ground coriander, smoked paprika, chili powder, salt, and pepper. Cook for another minute until fragrant.

4. Add diced tomatoes (with their juices) and tomato paste to the pot. Stir well to combine.

5. Pour in vegetable broth and bring the mixture to a simmer. Allow it to simmer for about 15-20 minutes, stirring occasionally, until the eggplant is tender and the flavors have melded together.

6. Add the drained and rinsed chickpeas to the stew. Stir to combine and cook for an additional 5-10 minutes to heat the chickpeas through.

7. Taste and adjust seasoning if needed. Once the stew is ready, remove it from heat. Serve the Eggplant and Chickpea Stew hot, garnished with chopped fresh parsley or cilantro.

8. Enjoy this delicious and satisfying stew on its own or with some crusty bread or rice for a complete meal!

This Eggplant and Chickpea Stew is packed with protein, fiber, and flavor, making it a perfect choice for a nutritious and filling meal. Feel free to customize the recipe by adding your favorite herbs, spices, or additional vegetables.

67. Grilled shrimp with a quinoa and vegetable salad

Ingredients:
- 1 pound large shrimp, peeled and deveined
- 2 tablespoons olive oil
- 2 cloves garlic, minced
- 1 teaspoon smoked paprika
- 1 teaspoon dried oregano
- Salt and pepper to taste
- Lemon wedges, for serving
- Skewers (if using wooden skewers, soak them in water for at least 30 minutes before grilling)

Instructions:
1. In a bowl, combine olive oil, minced garlic, smoked paprika, dried oregano, salt, and pepper. Mix well.

2. Add the peeled and deveined shrimp to the bowl and toss to coat them evenly with the marinade. Let the shrimp marinate for about 15-30 minutes in the refrigerator.

3. Preheat your grill to medium-high heat.

4. Thread the marinated shrimp onto skewers, leaving a little space between each shrimp.

5. Place the shrimp skewers on the preheated grill and cook for 2-3 minutes per side, or until they are pink and opaque.

6. Once the shrimp are cooked through, remove them from the grill and transfer them to a serving platter.

7. Serve the grilled shrimp hot, with lemon wedges on the side for squeezing over the shrimp.

Quinoa and Vegetable Salad:
Ingredients:
- 1 cup quinoa, rinsed
- 2 cups water or vegetable broth
- 1 red bell pepper, diced
- 1 yellow bell pepper, diced
- 1 cucumber, diced
- 1 cup cherry tomatoes, halved
- 1/4 cup red onion, finely chopped
- 1/4 cup fresh parsley, chopped
- 2 tablespoons fresh lemon juice
- 2 tablespoons olive oil
- Salt and pepper to taste

Instructions:

1. In a medium saucepan, bring the water or vegetable broth to a boil. Add the rinsed quinoa, reduce the heat to low, cover, and simmer for about 15 minutes, or until the quinoa is cooked and the liquid is absorbed. Remove from heat and let it cool slightly.

2. In a large bowl, combine the cooked quinoa, diced red and yellow bell peppers, diced cucumber, halved cherry tomatoes, finely chopped red onion, and chopped fresh parsley.

3. In a small bowl, whisk together the fresh lemon juice, olive oil, salt, and pepper to make the dressing.

4. Pour the dressing over the quinoa and vegetable mixture. Toss until everything is well coated.

5. Taste and adjust seasoning if needed.

6. Serve the quinoa and vegetable salad alongside the grilled shrimp.

7. Enjoy your delicious and nutritious meal!

This grilled shrimp with quinoa and vegetable salad is not only flavorful but also packed with protein, fiber, vitamins, and minerals. It's perfect for a light and satisfying lunch or dinner. Feel free to customize the salad with your favorite vegetables or add some avocado slices for extra creaminess.

68. Lentil and vegetable pasta

Ingredients:
- 1 can (14 oz) diced tomatoes
- 2 cups vegetable broth or water
- 1 teaspoon dried oregano
- 1 teaspoon dried basil
- 1/2 teaspoon red pepper
flakes (optional, for heat)
- Salt and pepper to taste
- Grated Parmesan cheese
 or nutritional yeast (for serving)
- Fresh parsley, chopped (for garnish)
- 8 oz (about 225g) pasta of your choice (such as penne, fusilli, or spaghetti)
- 1 cup dried lentils (green or brown), rinsed and drained
- 2 tablespoons olive oil
- 1 onion, diced
- 2 cloves garlic, minced
- 2 carrots, diced
- 2 celery stalks, diced
- 1 bell pepper, diced (any color)
- 1 zucchini, diced

Instructions:

1. Cook the pasta according to the package instructions until al dente. Drain and set aside.

2. While the pasta is cooking, heat olive oil in a large skillet or pot over medium heat.

3. Add diced onion and minced garlic to the skillet. Cook until the onion is soft and translucent, about 5 minutes.

4. Add diced carrots, celery, bell pepper, and zucchini to the skillet. Cook, stirring occasionally, for about 5-7 minutes, or until the vegetables are slightly softened.

5. Stir in dried oregano, dried basil, and red pepper flakes (if using). Season with salt and pepper to taste.

6. Add rinsed lentils, diced tomatoes (with their juices), and vegetable broth or water to the skillet. Stir well to combine.

7. Bring the mixture to a simmer, then reduce heat to low. Cover and cook for about 20-25 minutes, or until the lentils are tender and the sauce has thickened, stirring occasionally.

8. Once the lentils are cooked, add the cooked pasta to the skillet. Toss until the pasta is evenly coated with the lentil and vegetable mixture. Taste and adjust seasoning if needed.

9. Serve the Lentil and Vegetable Pasta hot, garnished with grated Parmesan cheese or nutritional yeast, and chopped fresh parsley. Enjoy your hearty and flavorful meal!

This Lentil and Vegetable Pasta is a great way to incorporate more plant-based protein and fiber into your diet. Feel free to customize the recipe by adding your favorite vegetables or herbs, or by using different types of pasta. It's a versatile dish that's perfect for weeknight dinners or meal prep.

69. Chicken and avocado wrap with whole grain tortilla

Ingredients:
- 2 whole grain tortillas (10-inch diameter)
- 1 cooked chicken breast, shredded or sliced
- 1 ripe avocado, sliced
- 1/2 cup cherry tomatoes, halved
- 1/4 cup red onion, thinly sliced
- 1/4 cup cucumber, thinly sliced
- 1/4 cup shredded lettuce or spinach leaves
- 2 tablespoons Greek yogurt or sour cream
- 1 tablespoon lime juice
- Salt and pepper to taste
- Hot sauce or salsa (optional, for added flavor)
- Fresh cilantro, chopped (for garnish)

Instructions:

1. In a small bowl, mix together Greek yogurt (or sour cream) with lime juice. Season with salt and pepper to taste. This will be the dressing for your wrap.

2. Lay the whole grain tortillas flat on a clean surface.

3. Divide the shredded chicken evenly between the two tortillas, placing it in the center of each tortilla.

4. Top the chicken with sliced avocado, halved cherry tomatoes, thinly sliced red onion, thinly sliced cucumber, and shredded lettuce or spinach leaves.

5. Drizzle the Greek yogurt dressing over the fillings on each tortilla.

6. If desired, add a few dashes of hot sauce or salsa for extra flavor.

7. Carefully fold the sides of the tortillas over the fillings, then roll them up tightly to form wraps.

8. Slice the wraps in half diagonally if desired, or serve them whole. Garnish with chopped fresh cilantro. Serve the Chicken and Avocado Wraps immediately, and enjoy!

These wraps are perfect for a quick lunch or dinner, and they're packed with protein, healthy fats, and fiber. Feel free to customize the fillings based on your preferences or what you have on hand. You can also make these wraps ahead of time for meal prep or on-the-go lunches. Enjoy!

70. Broiled sardines with a side of mixed greens

Broiled Sardines:
Ingredients:
- 4 fresh whole sardines, cleaned and gutted
- 2 tablespoons olive oil
- 2 cloves garlic, minced

- 1 teaspoon lemon zest
- 1 tablespoon lemon juice
- Salt and pepper to taste
- Fresh parsley, chopped (for garnish)
- Lemon wedges (for serving)

Instructions:
1. Preheat the broiler in your oven on high heat.

2. In a small bowl, mix together olive oil, minced garlic, lemon zest, lemon juice, salt, and pepper.

3. Place the cleaned and gutted sardines on a baking sheet lined with parchment paper or aluminum foil.

4. Brush the sardines generously with the olive oil mixture, making sure to coat both sides.

5. Place the baking sheet under the broiler and cook for about 3-4 minutes on each side, or until the sardines are cooked through and nicely browned.

6. Remove the sardines from the oven and transfer them to a serving platter. Garnish with chopped fresh parsley and serve with lemon wedges on the side.

Mixed Greens Salad:
Ingredients:
- 1/4 cup red onion, thinly sliced
- 2 tablespoons balsamic vinegar
- 2 tablespoons extra virgin olive oil

- 4 cups mixed salad greens (such as lettuce, spinach, arugula)
- Salt and pepper to taste
- 1/2 cup cherry tomatoes, halved
- 1/4 cup cucumber, sliced

Instructions:
1. In a large salad bowl, combine mixed salad greens, halved cherry tomatoes, sliced cucumber, and thinly sliced red onion.

2. In a small bowl, whisk together balsamic vinegar, extra virgin olive oil, salt, and pepper to make the dressing. Drizzle the dressing over the salad and toss until everything is well coated. Serve the mixed greens salad alongside the broiled sardines.

This dish is not only tasty but also rich in omega-3 fatty acids, protein, and essential nutrients from the sardines and mixed greens. It's a great option for a light and satisfying lunch or dinner.

71. Spinach and chickpea curry

Ingredients:
- 1 tablespoon oil
(such as olive oil or coconut oil)
- 1 onion, finely chopped
- 3 cloves garlic, minced
- 1-inch piece of ginger, grated
- 1 teaspoon cumin seeds
- 1 teaspoon ground coriander
- 1 teaspoon ground turmeric
- 1/2 teaspoon ground cayenne pepper (adjust to taste)
- 1 can (14 oz) diced tomatoes
- 1 can (14 oz) chickpeas, drained and rinsed
- 1 can (14 oz) coconut milk
- 1 lb fresh spinach leaves, washed and chopped
- Salt to taste
- Fresh cilantro, chopped (for garnish)
- Cooked rice or naan bread (for serving)

Instructions:

1. Heat oil in a large skillet or pot over medium heat. Add chopped onion and cook until softened, about 5 minutes.

2. Add minced garlic, grated ginger, and cumin seeds to the skillet. Cook for another 2 minutes until fragrant.

3. Stir in ground coriander, ground turmeric, and ground cayenne pepper. Cook for an additional minute.

4. Add diced tomatoes (with their juices) to the skillet. Stir well to combine.

5. Add drained and rinsed chickpeas to the skillet, stirring to coat them with the spices and tomatoes.

6. Pour in coconut milk and stir until everything is well combined. Bring the mixture to a simmer.

7. Once simmering, add chopped spinach leaves to the skillet in batches, stirring until wilted before adding more.

8. Allow the curry to simmer for about 10-15 minutes, stirring occasionally, until the flavors have melded together and the spinach is cooked down.

9. Taste the curry and adjust the seasoning with salt as needed. Once the curry is ready, remove it from heat. Serve the Spinach and Chickpea Curry hot, garnished with chopped fresh cilantro. Serve with cooked rice or naan bread on the side.

Enjoy your delicious and nutritious Spinach and Chickpea Curry! This dish is rich in protein, fiber, and essential nutrients, making it a satisfying vegetarian meal option. Feel free to adjust the spices and seasonings according to your taste preferences.

72. Roasted turkey breast with Brussels sprouts

Ingredients:

- 4 cloves garlic, minced
- 1 teaspoon dried thyme
- 1 teaspoon dried rosemary
- Salt and pepper to taste
- 1 lemon, sliced
- Fresh parsley, chopped (for garnish)

- 1 turkey breast (bone-in or boneless, depending on preference)
- 1 lb Brussels sprouts, trimmed and halved
- 3 tablespoons olive oil

Instructions:

1. Preheat your oven to 375°F (190°C).

2. If using a bone-in turkey breast, place it on a roasting rack set inside a roasting pan. If using a boneless turkey breast, you can place it directly in the roasting pan.

3. In a small bowl, mix together olive oil, minced garlic, dried thyme, dried rosemary, salt, and pepper.

4. Rub the olive oil mixture all over the turkey breast, making sure to coat it evenly.

5. Arrange the halved Brussels sprouts around the turkey breast in the roasting pan. Drizzle them with a little olive oil and season with salt and pepper.

6. Place lemon slices on top of the turkey breast.

7. Roast in the preheated oven for about 60-75 minutes, or until the internal temperature of the turkey breast reaches 165°F (74°C) and the Brussels sprouts are tender and caramelized, stirring the Brussels sprouts halfway through cooking.

8. Once done, remove the turkey breast from the oven and let it rest for about 10 minutes before slicing. Transfer the roasted Brussels sprouts to a serving platter.

10. Slice the roasted turkey breast and arrange it on the platter with the Brussels sprouts. Garnish with chopped fresh parsley for a pop of color and freshness. Serve hot and enjoy your delicious Roasted Turkey Breast with Brussels Sprouts!

Feel free to customize this recipe by adding your favorite herbs or spices to the turkey breast rub, or by adding other roasted vegetables alongside the Brussels sprouts. It's a versatile and satisfying meal that's sure to please a crowd.

73. Tofu and broccoli stir-fry with quinoa

Ingredients:
For the Tofu and Broccoli Stir-Fry:
- 14 oz (400g) firm tofu, pressed and cubed
- 2 tablespoons soy sauce (or tamari for gluten-free option)
- 1 tablespoon sesame oil
- 2 cloves garlic, minced
- 1 tablespoon ginger, minced
- 1 head broccoli, cut into florets
- 1 red bell pepper, sliced
- 1 carrot, julienned
- 4 green onions, chopped
- 2 tablespoons vegetable oil (for stir-frying)
- Sesame seeds for garnish (optional)

For the Quinoa:
- 1 cup quinoa, rinsed
- 2 cups water or vegetable broth
- Salt to taste

Instructions:
For the Quinoa:
1. In a medium saucepan, combine quinoa and water or vegetable broth.

2. Bring to a boil, then reduce heat to low, cover, and simmer for 15-20 minutes, or until quinoa is cooked and liquid is absorbed. Fluff the quinoa with a fork and season with salt to taste. Set aside.

For the Tofu and Broccoli Stir-Fry:
1. In a small bowl, combine cubed tofu with soy sauce and sesame oil. Let it marinate for 10-15 minutes.

2. Heat vegetable oil in a large skillet or wok over medium-high heat.

3. Add marinated tofu cubes to the skillet in a single layer. Cook for 3-4 minutes on each side, or until golden brown and crispy. Remove tofu from the skillet and set aside.

4. In the same skillet, add minced garlic and ginger. Cook for 1-2 minutes until fragrant.

5. Add broccoli florets, sliced red bell pepper, and julienned carrot to the skillet. Stir-fry for 4-5 minutes, or until vegetables are tender but still crisp.

6. Return the cooked tofu to the skillet. Add chopped green onions and toss everything together.

7. Cook for an additional 1-2 minutes, allowing the flavors to meld together.

8. Taste and adjust seasoning if needed.

To Serve:
1. Divide the cooked quinoa among serving bowls.

2. Top the quinoa with the tofu and broccoli stir-fry.

3. Garnish with sesame seeds if desired.

4. Serve hot and enjoy your delicious Tofu and Broccoli Stir-Fry with Quinoa!

This dish is not only tasty but also packed with protein, fiber, and nutrients. It's a satisfying and wholesome meal that's perfect for lunch or dinner. Feel free to customize the stir-fry with your favorite vegetables or add a dash of chili sauce for extra heat. Enjoy!

74. Kale and roasted beet salad with walnuts

Ingredients:
- 1 bunch kale, stems removed and leaves torn into bite-sized pieces
- 2 medium beets, roasted, peeled, and sliced
- 1/2 cup walnuts, toasted and chopped
- 1/4 cup crumbled feta cheese (optional, for added flavor)
- 2 tablespoons olive oil
- 1 tablespoon balsamic vinegar
- 1 tablespoon maple syrup (or honey)
- 1 teaspoon Dijon mustard
- Salt and pepper to taste
- 1/4 cup dried cranberries or raisins (optional, for sweetness)

Instructions:
For Roasting Beets:
1. Preheat your oven to 400°F (200°C).
2. Wash and trim the beets, leaving the skins on. Wrap each beet individually in aluminum foil.
3. Place the wrapped beets on a baking sheet and roast in the preheated oven for about 45-60 minutes, or until the beets are tender when pierced with a fork.
4. Once roasted, remove the beets from the oven and let them cool. Once cool enough to handle, peel off the skins and slice the beets into wedges or rounds. Set aside.

For the Salad:
1. In a small bowl, whisk together olive oil, balsamic vinegar, maple syrup (or honey), Dijon mustard, salt, and pepper to make the dressing.
2. Place torn kale leaves in a large salad bowl. Drizzle half of the dressing over the kale leaves.
3. Massage the kale leaves with your hands for a few minutes until they soften and become wilted.
4. Add roasted beet slices, toasted walnuts, and crumbled feta cheese (if using) to the bowl with the kale.
5. Add dried cranberries or raisins (if using) for a touch of sweetness.
6. Drizzle the remaining dressing over the salad and toss until everything is well coated.
7. Taste and adjust seasoning if needed.

To Serve:
1. Divide the kale and roasted beet salad among serving plates or bowls.
2. Garnish with additional toasted walnuts and crumbled feta cheese if desired.
3. Serve immediately and enjoy your delicious and nutritious Kale and Roasted Beet Salad with Walnuts

75. Quinoa and vegetable soup

Ingredients:
- 1 cup quinoa, rinsed
- 6 cups vegetable broth
- 1 onion, diced
- 2 carrots, diced
- 2 celery stalks, diced
- 3 cloves garlic, minced
- 1 bell pepper, diced
- 1 zucchini, diced
- 1 can (15 oz) chickpeas, drained and rinsed
- 2 teaspoons dried thyme
- 2 teaspoons dried oregano
- Salt and pepper to taste
- 1 can (14 oz) diced tomatoes
- 2 cups spinach leaves, chopped
- Fresh parsley, chopped (for garnish)
- Grated Parmesan cheese (optional, for serving)

Instructions:

1. In a large pot, combine quinoa and vegetable broth. Bring to a boil over medium-high heat.

2. Reduce heat to low, cover, and simmer for about 15 minutes, or until quinoa is cooked and tender.

3. In the meantime, heat a bit of olive oil in a separate skillet over medium heat. Add diced onion, carrots, celery, and minced garlic. Cook until vegetables are softened, about 5-7 minutes.

4. Add diced bell pepper and zucchini to the skillet. Cook for another 3-5 minutes, until the vegetables are tender-crisp.

5. Add the cooked vegetables to the pot with quinoa and vegetable broth.

6. Stir in diced tomatoes, drained and rinsed chickpeas, dried thyme, and dried oregano. Season with salt and pepper to taste.

7. Simmer the soup for an additional 10-15 minutes to allow the flavors to meld together. Stir in chopped spinach leaves and cook for another 2-3 minutes until wilted. Taste and adjust seasoning if needed.

8. Ladle the quinoa and vegetable soup into bowls. Garnish with chopped fresh parsley and grated Parmesan cheese if desired. Serve hot and enjoy your delicious and nutritious Quinoa and Vegetable Soup!

Feel free to customize this soup by adding your favorite vegetables or herbs. You can also swap out quinoa for other grains like rice or barley if you prefer. It's a versatile and satisfying dish that's perfect for meal prep or cozy weeknight dinners.

76. Grilled chicken with a side of roasted sweet potatoes

Grilled Chicken:
Ingredients:
- 4 boneless, skinless chicken breasts
- 2 tablespoons olive oil
- 2 cloves garlic, minced
- 1 teaspoon paprika
- 1 teaspoon dried oregano
- 1 teaspoon dried thyme
- Salt and pepper to taste

Instructions:
1. In a bowl, mix together the olive oil, minced garlic, paprika, oregano, thyme, salt, and pepper.
2. Place the chicken breasts in a shallow dish or a resealable plastic bag, and pour the marinade over them. Make sure the chicken is evenly coated. Marinate in the refrigerator for at least 30 minutes, or overnight for best results.
3. Preheat your grill to medium-high heat.
4. Remove the chicken from the marinade and discard any excess marinade.
5. Grill the chicken breasts for 6-8 minutes per side, or until they are cooked through and have reached an internal temperature of 165°F (75°C).
6. Once cooked, remove the chicken from the grill and let it rest for a few minutes before serving.

Roasted Sweet Potatoes:
Ingredients:
- 2 large sweet potatoes, peeled and cut into cubes
- 2 tablespoons olive oil
- 1 teaspoon garlic powder
- 1 teaspoon smoked paprika
- Salt and pepper to taste

Instructions:
1. Preheat your oven to 400°F (200°C).
2. In a large bowl, toss the sweet potato cubes with olive oil, garlic powder, smoked paprika, salt, and pepper until evenly coated.
3. Spread the sweet potatoes in a single layer on a baking sheet lined with parchment paper.
4. Roast in the preheated oven for 25-30 minutes, or until the sweet potatoes are tender and slightly caramelized, stirring halfway through cooking.
5. Once roasted, remove from the oven and serve alongside the grilled chicken.

77. Baked salmon with a side of steamed broccoli

Ingredients:
- 4 salmon fillets (about 6 oz each)
- Salt and pepper to taste
- Olive oil or cooking spray
- 1 lb broccoli florets
- Lemon wedges for serving (optional)

Instructions:
1. Preheat your oven to 400°F (200°C). Line a baking sheet with parchment paper or foil for easy cleanup.

2. Pat the salmon fillets dry with paper towels and season them with salt and pepper to taste on both sides.

3. Place the seasoned salmon fillets on the prepared baking sheet. Drizzle a little olive oil over the top of each fillet or spray them lightly with cooking spray.

4. Bake the salmon in the preheated oven for about 12-15 minutes, or until the salmon is cooked through and flakes easily with a fork.

5. While the salmon is baking, prepare the broccoli. Steam the broccoli florets in a steamer basket or in a pot with a little water until tender but still crisp, about 5-7 minutes.

6. Once the salmon is done, remove it from the oven and let it rest for a few minutes.

7. Serve the baked salmon hot with a side of steamed broccoli.

8. Garnish with lemon wedges if desired, for an extra burst of flavor.

9. Enjoy this simple and nutritious meal of Baked Salmon with Steamed Broccoli!

Feel free to customize the seasoning of the salmon with your favorite herbs and spices, or drizzle some lemon juice over the top before serving for added freshness.

78. Chickpea and tomato stew

Ingredients:
- 2 tablespoons olive oil
- 1 onion, chopped
- 3 cloves garlic, minced
- 1 teaspoon ground cumin
- 1 teaspoon ground paprika
- 1/2 teaspoon ground turmeric
- 1 can (14 oz) diced tomatoes
- 2 cans (14 oz each) chickpeas, drained and rinsed
- 2 cups vegetable broth
- Salt and pepper to taste
- Fresh parsley or cilantro, chopped, for garnish (optional)

Instructions:
1. Heat the olive oil in a large pot over medium heat.

2. Add the chopped onion to the pot and cook until softened, about 5 minutes.

3. Stir in the minced garlic, ground cumin, ground paprika, and ground turmeric. Cook for another 1-2 minutes until fragrant.

4. Add the diced tomatoes (with their juices) to the pot, along with the drained and rinsed chickpeas.

5. Pour in the vegetable broth and stir to combine.

6. Bring the stew to a simmer, then reduce the heat to low. Cover and let it simmer for about 15-20 minutes to allow the flavors to meld together and the stew to thicken slightly.

7. Taste and season the stew with salt and pepper as needed.

8. Once done, remove the pot from the heat and let the stew cool slightly before serving. Garnish the Chickpea and Tomato Stew with chopped fresh parsley or cilantro if desired.

9. Serve the stew hot as a comforting and satisfying meal. Enjoy the delicious flavors and textures of this simple and nutritious Chickpea and Tomato Stew!

Feel free to customize the stew by adding other vegetables such as spinach, kale, or bell peppers, or by incorporating spices like chili powder or smoked paprika for extra depth of flavor.

79. Lentil and vegetable stuffed bell peppers

Ingredients:
- 4 large bell peppers, any color
- 1 cup dry lentils (green or brown), rinsed
- 2 cups vegetable broth or water
- 1 tablespoon olive oil
- 1 onion, diced
- 2 cloves garlic, minced
- 1 carrot, diced
- 1 zucchini, diced
- 1 cup diced tomatoes (fresh or canned)
- 1 teaspoon dried thyme
- 1 teaspoon dried oregano
- Salt and pepper to taste
- Grated cheese for topping (optional)
- Fresh parsley or basil, chopped, for garnish (optional)

Instructions:
1. Preheat your oven to 375°F (190°C).
Cut the tops off the bell peppers and remove the seeds and membranes.

2. In a medium saucepan, bring the vegetable broth or water to a boil. Add the lentils, reduce the heat to low, cover, and simmer for about 20-25 minutes, or until the lentils are tender and the liquid is absorbed. Remove from heat and set aside.

3. In a large skillet, heat the olive oil over medium heat. Add the diced onion and cook until softened, about 3-4 minutes.

4. Add the minced garlic to the skillet and cook for another minute until fragrant.

5. Stir in the diced carrot and zucchini, and cook for about 5 minutes, or until they start to soften.

6. Add the diced tomatoes, dried thyme, dried oregano, cooked lentils, salt, and pepper to the skillet. Stir until well combined and heated through. Adjust seasoning to taste.

7. Spoon the lentil and vegetable mixture into the hollowed-out bell peppers, pressing it down gently to pack it in.

8. Place the stuffed bell peppers in a baking dish, standing upright. Cover the baking dish with aluminum foil and bake in the preheated oven for about 25-30 minutes, or until the bell peppers are tender.

9. If using, sprinkle grated cheese over the top of each stuffed bell pepper during the last 5 minutes of baking.

10. Once done, remove the stuffed bell peppers from the oven and let them cool for a minute. Garnish with chopped fresh parsley or basil if desired. Serve the Lentil and Vegetable Stuffed Bell Peppers hot as a delicious and satisfying meal.

80. Baked tilapia with a side of green beans

Ingredients:
- 4 tilapia fillets
- Salt and pepper to taste
- Olive oil or cooking spray
- 1 lb fresh green beans, trimmed
- Lemon wedges for serving (optional)
- Fresh parsley, chopped, for garnish (optional)

Instructions:
1. Preheat your oven to 400°F (200°C). Line a baking sheet with parchment paper or foil for easy cleanup.

2. Pat the tilapia fillets dry with paper towels and season them with salt and pepper to taste on both sides.

3. Place the seasoned tilapia fillets on the prepared baking sheet. Drizzle a little olive oil over the top of each fillet or spray them lightly with cooking spray.

4. Bake the tilapia in the preheated oven for about 12-15 minutes, or until the fish is cooked through and flakes easily with a fork.

5. While the tilapia is baking, prepare the green beans. Steam or boil the green beans in a pot of salted water until tender but still crisp, about 5-7 minutes. Drain and set aside.

6. Once the tilapia is done, remove it from the oven and let it rest for a few minutes.

7. Serve the baked tilapia hot with a side of steamed green beans.

8. Garnish with lemon wedges and chopped fresh parsley if desired, for an extra burst of flavor.

9. Enjoy this simple and nutritious meal of Baked Tilapia with Green Beans!

Feel free to customize the seasoning of the tilapia with your favorite herbs and spices, or drizzle some lemon juice over the top before serving for added freshness.

81. Grilled vegetable and tofu skewers

Ingredients:
- 1/4 cup olive oil
- 2 tablespoons balsamic vinegar
- 2 cloves garlic, minced
- 1 teaspoon dried herbs
(such as thyme, oregano, or basil)
- Salt and pepper to taste
- Wooden or metal skewers

- 1 block (14 oz) extra firm tofu, pressed
and cut into cubes
- 2 bell peppers, any color, cut into chunks
- 1 zucchini, sliced into rounds
- 1 yellow squash, sliced into rounds
- 1 red onion, cut into chunks
- Cherry tomatoes

Instructions:

1. If using wooden skewers, soak them in water for at least 30 minutes to prevent burning.

2. In a small bowl, whisk together the olive oil, balsamic vinegar, minced garlic, dried herbs, salt, and pepper to make the marinade.

3. Place the tofu cubes in a shallow dish and pour half of the marinade over them. Toss to coat evenly and let them marinate for at least 30 minutes, or longer if possible, in the refrigerator.

4. Preheat your grill to medium-high heat.

5. Thread the marinated tofu cubes and prepared vegetables onto the skewers, alternating between tofu and vegetables. Brush the skewers with the remaining marinade.

7. Place the skewers on the preheated grill and cook for about 8-10 minutes, turning occasionally, until the vegetables are tender and the tofu is lightly browned and crispy on the edges.

8. Once done, remove the skewers from the grill and transfer them to a serving platter.

9. Serve the Grilled Vegetable and Tofu Skewers hot, accompanied by your favorite dipping sauce or served over cooked rice or quinoa.

10. Enjoy the delicious flavors of these grilled skewers, packed with nutritious vegetables and protein-rich tofu!

Feel free to customize the vegetables according to your preference or what's in season. You can also add mushrooms, cherry tomatoes, or chunks of pineapple for extra flavor and variety.

82. Spinach and lentil soup

Ingredients:
- 1 cup dried green or brown lentils, rinsed
- 1 tablespoon olive oil
- 1 onion, chopped
- 2 cloves garlic, minced
- 2 carrots, diced
- 2 celery stalks, diced
- 6 cups vegetable broth or water
- 1 can (14 oz) diced tomatoes
- 2 cups fresh spinach, chopped
- 1 teaspoon dried thyme
- 1 teaspoon dried oregano
- Salt and pepper to taste
- Lemon wedges for serving (optional)
- Grated Parmesan cheese for serving (optional)

Instructions:
1. In a large pot, heat the olive oil over medium heat. Add the chopped onion and cook until softened, about 5 minutes.

2. Add the minced garlic, diced carrots, and diced celery to the pot. Cook for another 3-4 minutes, stirring occasionally.

3. Stir in the rinsed lentils, vegetable broth or water, diced tomatoes (with their juices), dried thyme, and dried oregano. Bring the soup to a boil.

4. Reduce the heat to low, cover the pot, and let the soup simmer for about 20-25 minutes, or until the lentils are tender.

5. Stir in the chopped spinach and cook for another 2-3 minutes, or until the spinach is wilted.

6. Taste the soup and season with salt and pepper as needed. Once done, remove the pot from the heat. Ladle the Spinach and Lentil Soup into bowls.

7. Serve hot, garnished with lemon wedges and grated Parmesan cheese if desired.Enjoy the warm and comforting flavors of this nutritious Spinach and Lentil Soup!

Feel free to customize the soup by adding other vegetables such as diced potatoes, chopped kale, or sliced mushrooms. You can also add a dash of hot sauce or sprinkle of red pepper flakes for some heat.

83. Quinoa and black bean burgers

Ingredients:
- 1 cup cooked quinoa
- 1 can (15 oz) black beans, drained and rinsed
- 1/2 cup breadcrumbs (or almond meal for gluten-free option)
- 1/4 cup finely chopped onion
- 2 cloves garlic, minced
- 1 teaspoon ground cumin
- 1 teaspoon chili powder
- 1/2 teaspoon paprika
- Salt and pepper to taste
- 1 egg, beaten (or flaxseed egg for vegan option)
- 2 tablespoons olive oil, for cooking

Instructions:
1. In a large mixing bowl, mash the black beans with a fork or potato masher until mostly smooth, leaving some beans intact for texture.

2. Add the cooked quinoa, breadcrumbs, finely chopped onion, minced garlic, ground cumin, chili powder, paprika, salt, and pepper to the bowl. Mix until well combined.

3. Add the beaten egg to the mixture and stir until everything is evenly incorporated. If the mixture is too wet, add more breadcrumbs as needed.

4. Divide the mixture into 4-6 portions, depending on how large you want your burgers to be. Shape each portion into a patty.

5. Heat the olive oil in a large skillet over medium heat.

6. Once the oil is hot, add the quinoa and black bean patties to the skillet. Cook for about 4-5 minutes on each side, or until golden brown and crispy.

7. Once done, remove the patties from the skillet and let them cool slightly.

8. Serve the Quinoa and Black Bean Burgers on burger buns with your favorite toppings such as lettuce, tomato, avocado, onion, and condiments. Enjoy these delicious and protein-packed burgers as a satisfying and nutritious meal!

Feel free to customize the recipe by adding other ingredients such as grated carrots, bell peppers, or fresh herbs. You can also bake the burgers in the oven instead of frying them for a healthier option.

84. Broiled trout with a side of roasted Brussels sprouts

Ingredients:
- 4 trout fillets
- Salt and pepper to taste
- Olive oil
- 1 lb Brussels sprouts, trimmed and halved
- 2 tablespoons balsamic vinegar
- 2 tablespoons honey or maple syrup
- 2 cloves garlic, minced
- 2 tablespoons olive oil
- Salt and pepper to taste
- Lemon wedges for serving

Instructions:
For the Broiled Trout:
1. Preheat the broiler in your oven.
2. Season the trout fillets with salt and pepper on both sides.
3. Place the seasoned trout fillets on a baking sheet lined with aluminum foil.
4. Drizzle olive oil over the trout fillets.
5. Place the baking sheet under the broiler and cook for about 4-6 minutes on each side, or until the fish is cooked through and flakes easily with a fork.
6. Once done, remove the trout from the oven and set aside.

For the Roasted Brussels Sprouts:
1. Preheat your oven to 400°F (200°C).
2. In a large bowl, whisk together balsamic vinegar, honey or maple syrup, minced garlic, olive oil, salt, and pepper.
3. Add the trimmed and halved Brussels sprouts to the bowl and toss until they are evenly coated with the marinade.
4. Spread the Brussels sprouts out in a single layer on a baking sheet lined with parchment paper or foil.
5. Roast in the preheated oven for about 20-25 minutes, or until the Brussels sprouts are tender and caramelized, stirring halfway through to ensure even cooking. Once done, remove the roasted Brussels sprouts from the oven.

Serving: Serve the broiled trout fillets hot with a side of roasted Brussels sprouts. Garnish with lemon wedges for a fresh burst of flavor.Enjoy this flavorful and nutritious meal!

Feel free to customize the seasoning of the trout with your favorite herbs and spices, or add lemon slices on top of the fillets before broiling for extra zest. You can also sprinkle some grated Parmesan cheese over the roasted Brussels sprouts before serving for added richness.

85. Cauliflower and chickpea tacos

Ingredients:
- 1 head cauliflower, cut into florets
- 1 can (15 oz) chickpeas, drained and rinsed
- 2 tablespoons olive oil
- 1 teaspoon chili powder
- 1 teaspoon ground cumin
- 1/2 teaspoon smoked paprika
- 1/2 teaspoon garlic powder
- Salt and pepper to taste
- 8 small tortillas (corn or flour)
- Toppings of your choice: shredded lettuce, diced tomatoes, diced avocado, sliced red onion, salsa, sour cream, lime wedges, etc.

Instructions:
1. Preheat your oven to 400°F (200°C).

2. In a large mixing bowl, toss the cauliflower florets and chickpeas with olive oil, chili powder, ground cumin, smoked paprika, garlic powder, salt, and pepper until evenly coated.

3. Spread the seasoned cauliflower and chickpeas out in a single layer on a baking sheet lined with parchment paper or foil.

4. Roast in the preheated oven for about 20-25 minutes, or until the cauliflower is tender and lightly browned, and the chickpeas are crispy, stirring halfway through.

5. While the cauliflower and chickpeas are roasting, warm the tortillas according to package instructions.

6. Once done, remove the baking sheet from the oven.

7. Assemble the tacos by filling each tortilla with roasted cauliflower and chickpeas, and your desired toppings.

8. Squeeze some lime juice over the top if desired, for extra freshness.

9. Serve the Cauliflower and Chickpea Tacos hot and enjoy!

Feel free to customize your tacos with additional toppings such as shredded cheese, salsa verde, cilantro, or pickled jalapeños. You can also drizzle some creamy chipotle sauce or tahini dressing over the filling for extra flavor.

86. Chicken and vegetable stir-fry with brown rice

Ingredients:
- 2 boneless, skinless chicken breasts, thinly sliced
- 2 tablespoons soy sauce
- 1 tablespoon cornstarch
- 2 tablespoons vegetable oil, divided
- 2 cups mixed vegetables (such as bell peppers, broccoli, carrots, snap peas)
- 3 cloves garlic, minced
- 1 tablespoon minced ginger
- Cooked brown rice, for serving

For the sauce:
- 1/4 cup soy sauce
- 2 tablespoons oyster sauce
- 1 tablespoon hoisin sauce
- 1 teaspoon sesame oil
- 1 teaspoon cornstarch

Instructions:
1. In a small bowl, mix together 2 tablespoons of soy sauce and 1 tablespoon of cornstarch. Add the sliced chicken breasts and toss to coat. Let it marinate for about 15 minutes.

2. In another small bowl, whisk together all the ingredients for the sauce: soy sauce, oyster sauce, hoisin sauce, sesame oil, and cornstarch. Set aside.

3. Heat 1 tablespoon of vegetable oil in a large skillet or wok over medium-high heat. Add the marinated chicken and stir-fry until cooked through, about 5-6 minutes. Remove the chicken from the skillet and set aside.

4. In the same skillet, add the remaining tablespoon of vegetable oil. Add the mixed vegetables and stir-fry for about 3-4 minutes, or until they are tender-crisp.

5. Add the minced garlic and ginger to the skillet and cook for another 1-2 minutes, until fragrant.

6. Return the cooked chicken to the skillet. Pour the sauce over the chicken and vegetables. Stir everything together and cook for another 1-2 minutes, or until the sauce has thickened slightly.

7. Serve the chicken and vegetable stir-fry hot over cooked brown rice. Enjoy your delicious and nutritious Chicken and Vegetable Stir-Fry with Brown Rice

87. Grilled mackerel with a side of steamed spinach

Ingredients:
- 4 mackerel fillets
- Salt and pepper to taste
- Olive oil
- Lemon wedges for serving (optional)
- Fresh parsley, chopped, for garnish (optional)
- 1 lb fresh spinach leaves, washed and trimmed
- 2 cloves garlic, minced
- 1 tablespoon olive oil
- Salt and pepper to taste

Instructions:
For the Grilled Mackerel:
1. Preheat your grill to medium-high heat.
2. Pat the mackerel fillets dry with paper towels.
3. Season both sides of the mackerel fillets with salt, pepper, and a drizzle of olive oil.
4. Place the seasoned mackerel fillets on the preheated grill and cook for about 3-4 minutes on each side, or until the fish is cooked through and easily flakes with a fork.
5. Once done, remove the grilled mackerel from the grill and set aside.

For the Steamed Spinach:
1. In a large skillet or pot, heat 1 tablespoon of olive oil over medium heat.
2. Add the minced garlic to the skillet and cook for about 1 minute, or until fragrant.
3. Add the fresh spinach leaves to the skillet. You may need to do this in batches, adding more spinach as it wilts down.
4. Cover the skillet and let the spinach steam for about 2-3 minutes, or until wilted.
5. Once the spinach is wilted, remove the skillet from the heat.
6. Season the steamed spinach with salt and pepper to taste.

Serving:
1. Serve the Grilled Mackerel hot with a side of Steamed Spinach.
2. Garnish with lemon wedges and chopped fresh parsley if desired.
3. Enjoy this flavorful and nutritious meal!

Feel free to add other seasonings or herbs to the mackerel before grilling for extra flavor. You can also drizzle some lemon juice over the grilled mackerel before serving for a fresh citrusy touch.

88. Eggplant and lentil stew

Ingredients:
- 1 large eggplant, diced
- 1 cup dried green or brown lentils, rinsed
- 1 onion, chopped
- 2 cloves garlic, minced
- 1 can (14 oz) diced tomatoes
- 4 cups vegetable broth
- 1 teaspoon ground cumin
- 1 teaspoon paprika
- 1/2 teaspoon dried thyme
- Salt and pepper to taste
- Olive oil for cooking
- Fresh parsley or cilantro, chopped, for garnish (optional)

Instructions:

1. In a large pot or Dutch oven, heat a drizzle of olive oil over medium heat. Add the chopped onion and minced garlic, and cook until softened and fragrant, about 5 minutes.

2. Add the diced eggplant to the pot and cook for another 5 minutes, stirring occasionally, until it starts to soften.

3. Stir in the rinsed lentils, diced tomatoes (with their juices), vegetable broth, ground cumin, paprika, dried thyme, salt, and pepper.

4. Bring the stew to a boil, then reduce the heat to low. Cover and let it simmer for about 20-25 minutes, or until the lentils are tender and the stew has thickened.

5. Once done, taste the stew and adjust the seasoning if needed.

6. Serve the Eggplant and Lentil Stew hot, garnished with chopped fresh parsley or cilantro if desired.

7. Enjoy this hearty and flavorful stew as a comforting meal!

Feel free to customize the stew by adding other vegetables such as diced bell peppers, carrots, or zucchini. You can also add a splash of balsamic vinegar or a sprinkle of red pepper flakes for extra flavor.

89. Tofu and vegetable kebabs with quinoa

Ingredients:
- 2 tablespoons soy sauce
- 2 cloves garlic, minced
- 1 teaspoon ground ginger
- 1 teaspoon honey or maple syrup
- Salt and pepper to taste
- Cooked quinoa, for serving
- Wooden or metal skewers

- 1 block (14 oz) extra firm tofu, pressed and cubed
- 2 bell peppers, any color, cut into chunks
- 1 zucchini, sliced into rounds
- 1 red onion, cut into chunks
- Cherry tomatoes
- 2 tablespoons olive oil

Instructions:
1. If using wooden skewers, soak them in water for at least 30 minutes to prevent burning.

2. In a small bowl, whisk together the olive oil, soy sauce, minced garlic, ground ginger, honey or maple syrup, salt, and pepper to make the marinade.

3. Place the cubed tofu, bell pepper chunks, zucchini slices, red onion chunks, and cherry tomatoes in a large mixing bowl. Pour the marinade over the tofu and vegetables, and toss until evenly coated. Let them marinate for about 15-30 minutes.

4. Preheat your grill or grill pan to medium-high heat.

5. Thread the marinated tofu cubes and vegetables onto the skewers, alternating between tofu and vegetables.

6. Brush any remaining marinade over the skewers.

7. Place the tofu and vegetable kebabs on the preheated grill or grill pan. Cook for about 8-10 minutes, turning occasionally, until the vegetables are tender and slightly charred, and the tofu is lightly browned.

8. Once done, remove the kebabs from the grill. Serve the Tofu and Vegetable Kebabs hot with cooked quinoa. Enjoy this flavorful and satisfying meal!

Feel free to customize the kebabs by adding other vegetables such as mushrooms, cherry tomatoes, or chunks of pineapple. You can also sprinkle some sesame seeds or chopped fresh herbs over the kebabs before serving for extra flavor and garnish.

90. Spinach and avocado smoothie

Ingredients:
- 1 ripe avocado, peeled and pitted
- 1 cup fresh spinach leaves
- 1 ripe banana, peeled
- 1 cup milk of your choice (such as almond milk, soy milk, or dairy milk)
- 1 tablespoon honey or maple syrup (optional, for sweetness)
- Ice cubes (optional, for a colder smoothie)

Instructions:
1. Place the peeled and pitted avocado, fresh spinach leaves, peeled banana, milk of your choice, and honey or maple syrup (if using) in a blender.

2. If you prefer a colder smoothie, add a handful of ice cubes to the blender as well.

3. Blend all the ingredients until smooth and creamy. If the smoothie is too thick, you can add more milk to reach your desired consistency.

4. Taste the smoothie and adjust the sweetness if needed by adding more honey or maple syrup.

5. Once blended to your liking, pour the Spinach and Avocado Smoothie into glasses.

6. Serve immediately and enjoy your nutritious and delicious smoothie!

Feel free to customize your smoothie by adding other ingredients such as protein powder, chia seeds, flaxseeds, or a splash of lime juice for extra flavor and nutrition. You can also substitute the banana with other fruits like mango, pineapple, or berries, depending on your preference.

91. Chickpea and vegetable curry with brown rice

Ingredients:
- 1 can (15 oz) chickpeas,
  drained and rinsed
- 1 tablespoon vegetable oil
- 1 onion, chopped
- 2 cloves garlic, minced
- 1 tablespoon grated ginger
- 2 teaspoons curry powder
- 1 teaspoon ground cumin
- 1 teaspoon ground coriander
- 1/2 teaspoon turmeric
- 1/4 teaspoon cayenne pepper (optional, for heat)
- 1 can (14 oz) diced tomatoes
- 1 can (14 oz) coconut milk
- 2 cups mixed vegetables (such as bell peppers, carrots, zucchini, peas)
- Salt and pepper to taste
- Cooked brown rice, for serving
- Fresh cilantro, chopped, for garnish (optional)
- Lime wedges for serving (optional)

Instructions:
1. Heat the vegetable oil in a large skillet or pot over medium heat. Add the chopped onion and cook until softened, about 5 minutes.

2. Add the minced garlic and grated ginger to the skillet, and cook for another minute until fragrant.

3. Stir in the curry powder, ground cumin, ground coriander, turmeric, and cayenne pepper (if using). Cook for another minute to toast the spices.

4. Add the diced tomatoes (with their juices), drained and rinsed chickpeas, coconut milk, and mixed vegetables to the skillet. Stir to combine.

5. Bring the mixture to a simmer, then reduce the heat to low. Cover and let it simmer for about 15-20 minutes, stirring occasionally, until the vegetables are tender and the flavors have melded together.

6. Taste the curry and adjust the seasoning with salt and pepper as needed. Once done, remove the skillet from the heat. Serve the Chickpea and Vegetable Curry hot over cooked brown rice.

7. Garnish with chopped fresh cilantro and serve with lime wedges on the side for squeezing over the curry if desired. Enjoy this flavorful and satisfying Chickpea and Vegetable Curry with Brown Rice!

Feel free to customize the curry by adding other vegetables or protein sources such as spinach, potatoes, cauliflower, or tofu. Adjust the level of spice according to your preference by adding more or less cayenne pepper.

92. Roasted chicken with a side of sweet potato mash

Ingredients:
- 4 bone-in, skin-on chicken thighs or breasts
- Salt, pepper, olive oil, paprika, dried thyme, garlic powder
- 1 lemon (optional)
- 2 large sweet potatoes, peeled and cubed
- 2 tbsp butter or olive oil
- 1/4 cup milk or cream
- Optional: maple syrup, cinnamon, nutmeg

Instructions:
1. Preheat oven to 400°F (200°C). Season chicken with salt, pepper, olive oil, paprika, thyme, and garlic powder. Roast for 25-30 min (thighs) or 30-35 min (breasts).

2. Boil sweet potatoes until fork-tender, then drain and mash with butter, milk/cream, salt, and pepper. Add optional ingredients if desired.

3. Serve roasted chicken with sweet potato mash.

4. Enjoy your comforting meal!

93. Grilled shrimp with a quinoa and kale salad

Ingredients:
- Shrimp
- Quinoa
- Kale
- Olive oil
- Lemon juice
- Garlic
- Salt and pepper
- Optional: cherry tomatoes, cucumber, feta cheese

Instructions:
1. Marinate shrimp in olive oil, lemon juice, garlic, salt, and pepper. Grill until cooked.

2. Cook quinoa according to package instructions.

3. Massage kale with olive oil and lemon juice to soften. Toss with cooked quinoa.

4. Optional: Add cherry tomatoes, cucumber, and feta cheese.

5. Serve grilled shrimp alongside quinoa and kale salad.

6. Enjoy your flavorful and nutritious meal!

94. Lentil and vegetable chili

Ingredients:
- 1 cup dried lentils
- 1 onion, chopped
- 2 cloves garlic, minced
- 2 carrots, diced
- 2 celery stalks, diced
- 1 bell pepper, diced
- 1 can (14 oz) diced tomatoes
- 1 can (14 oz) tomato sauce
- 2 cups vegetable broth
- 2 tablespoons chili powder
- 1 teaspoon ground cumin
- Salt and pepper to taste
- Olive oil

Instructions:
1. Rinse lentils and set aside.

2. In a large pot, sauté onion and garlic in olive oil until softened.

3. Add carrots, celery, bell pepper, and sauté until tender.

4. Stir in diced tomatoes, tomato sauce, vegetable broth, lentils, chili powder, cumin, salt, and pepper.

5. Bring to a boil, then reduce heat and simmer for 20-25 minutes until lentils are cooked and flavors are melded.

6. Adjust seasoning if needed.

7. Serve hot.

8. Enjoy your hearty Lentil and Vegetable Chili!

95. Baked salmon with a side of roasted asparagus

Ingredients:
- Salmon fillets
- Asparagus spears
- Olive oil
- Salt and pepper
- Lemon wedges (optional)

Instructions:
1. Preheat oven to 400°F (200°C).

2. Place salmon fillets on a baking sheet lined with parchment paper.

3. Drizzle salmon with olive oil and season with salt and pepper.

4. Trim asparagus spears and place them on another baking sheet.

5. Drizzle asparagus with olive oil and season with salt and pepper.

6. Bake both salmon and asparagus in the preheated oven for 12-15 minutes, or until salmon is cooked through and asparagus is tender.

7. Serve salmon hot with roasted asparagus.

8. Optionally, garnish with lemon wedges for extra flavor.

9. Enjoy your delicious and healthy meal!

96. Turkey and vegetable pasta

Ingredients:
- 8 oz pasta (of your choice)
- 1 lb ground turkey
- 2 cups mixed vegetables (such as bell peppers, zucchini, carrots)
- 2 cloves garlic, minced
- 1 can (14 oz) diced tomatoes
- 1 tablespoon tomato paste
- 1 teaspoon Italian seasoning
- Salt and pepper to taste
- Olive oil
- Grated Parmesan cheese for serving (optional)
- Fresh basil for garnish (optional)

Instructions:
1. Cook pasta according to package instructions. Drain and set aside.

2. In a large skillet, heat olive oil over medium heat. Add minced garlic and cook until fragrant.

3. Add ground turkey to the skillet and cook until browned, breaking it up with a spatula.

4. Stir in mixed vegetables and cook until softened.

5. Add diced tomatoes, tomato paste, Italian seasoning, salt, and pepper. Stir to combine.

6. Simmer for a few minutes until the flavors meld together.

7. Add cooked pasta to the skillet and toss to coat with the sauce.

8. Serve hot, optionally garnished with grated Parmesan cheese and fresh basil.

9. Enjoy your tasty Turkey and Vegetable Pasta!

97. Grilled chicken with a side of steamed broccoli

Ingredients:
- Chicken breasts
- Broccoli florets
- Olive oil
- Salt and pepper
- Lemon wedges (optional)

Instructions:
1. Preheat grill to medium-high heat.

2. Season chicken breasts with salt, pepper, and a drizzle of olive oil.

3. Grill chicken for 6-8 minutes per side, or until cooked through.

4. While chicken is grilling, steam broccoli until tender-crisp.

5. Serve grilled chicken hot with steamed broccoli.

6. Optionally, garnish with lemon wedges for extra flavor.

7. Enjoy your simple and nutritious meal!

98. Spinach and chickpea salad

Ingredients:
- 4 cups fresh spinach leaves
- 1 can (15 oz) chickpeas, drained and rinsed
- 1/2 red onion, thinly sliced
- 1/4 cup crumbled feta cheese (optional)
- 2 tablespoons olive oil
- 1 tablespoon balsamic vinegar
- 1 teaspoon Dijon mustard
- Salt and pepper to taste

Instructions:
1. In a large mixing bowl, combine the fresh spinach leaves, chickpeas, thinly sliced red onion, and crumbled feta cheese (if using).

2. In a small bowl, whisk together the olive oil, balsamic vinegar, Dijon mustard, salt, and pepper to make the dressing.

3. Pour the dressing over the salad and toss until everything is evenly coated.

4. Serve immediately or refrigerate until ready to serve.

5. Enjoy your refreshing Spinach and Chickpea Salad as a healthy and satisfying meal or side dish!

Feel free to customize your salad by adding other ingredients such as cherry tomatoes, cucumber slices, roasted bell peppers, or avocado slices. You can also sprinkle some toasted nuts or seeds on top for extra crunch.

99. Tofu and vegetable curry with quinoa

Ingredients:
- 2 tablespoons curry powder
- 1 teaspoon ground turmeric
- Salt and pepper to taste
- Cooked quinoa, for serving
- Fresh cilantro, chopped, for garnish (optional)
- Lime wedges, for serving (optional)

- 1 block (14 oz) firm tofu, cubed
- 2 cups mixed vegetables (such as bell peppers, carrots, broccoli)
- 1 onion, chopped
- 2 cloves garlic, minced
- 1 tablespoon grated ginger
- 1 can (14 oz) coconut milk
- 1 can (14 oz) diced tomatoes

Instructions:

1. In a large skillet or pot, heat some oil over medium heat. Add chopped onion and cook until softened.

2. Add minced garlic and grated ginger to the skillet and cook for another minute until fragrant.

3. Stir in curry powder and ground turmeric, and cook for another minute to toast the spices.

4. Add cubed tofu and mixed vegetables to the skillet, and cook for a few minutes until vegetables start to soften.

5. Pour in coconut milk and diced tomatoes (with their juices), and season with salt and pepper.

6. Simmer the curry for about 10-15 minutes, or until the vegetables are tender and the flavors are well combined.

7. Adjust seasoning if needed.Serve the tofu and vegetable curry hot over cooked quinoa.

8. Garnish with chopped fresh cilantro and serve with lime wedges on the side for squeezing over the curry if desired. Enjoy your delicious Tofu and Vegetable Curry with Quinoa!

Feel free to add other vegetables or protein sources such as spinach, potatoes, cauliflower, or chickpeas. You can also adjust the level of spice according to your preference by adding more or less curry powder.

100. Baked cod with a side of roasted carrots

Ingredients:
- 4 cod fillets
- 1 lb carrots, peeled and sliced into sticks
- Olive oil
- Salt and pepper
- Lemon wedges (optional)
- Fresh parsley, chopped, for garnish (optional)

Instructions:
1. Preheat your oven to 400°F (200°C).

2. Place the cod fillets on a baking sheet lined with parchment paper.

3. Drizzle olive oil over the cod fillets and season with salt and pepper.

4. Toss the carrot sticks with olive oil, salt, and pepper, and spread them out on another baking sheet.

5. Bake both the cod and carrots in the preheated oven for about 15-20 minutes, or until the cod is opaque and flakes easily with a fork, and the carrots are tender and caramelized.

6. Once done, remove the baking sheets from the oven.

7. Serve the baked cod hot with a side of roasted carrots.

8. Optionally, garnish with fresh parsley and serve with lemon wedges on the side for squeezing over the cod.

9. Enjoy your flavorful and nutritious Baked Cod with Roasted Carrots!

Feel free to customize your baked cod by adding herbs or spices such as dill, parsley, or paprika before baking. You can also add a squeeze of lemon juice over the cod before serving for extra brightness.

*As we conclude our journey through **"The Psoriatic Arthritis Diet Cookbook: 100+ Recipes for Happy Joints",** we hope you feel empowered and inspired to take control of your health and well-being through the power of nutrition. This cookbook has been carefully crafted to provide you with delicious recipes and valuable insights that support your journey towards managing psoriatic arthritis and promoting joint health.*

By incorporating anti-inflammatory ingredients and mindful eating habits into your diet, you have the opportunity to soothe inflammation, alleviate symptoms, and enhance your overall quality of life. The recipes in this book are not only nutritious and flavorful but also designed to be gentle on your joints, making it easier for you to enjoy delicious meals while supporting your health goals.

We understand that managing psoriatic arthritis can be challenging, but we hope this cookbook has provided you with practical tools and resources to navigate your journey with confidence. Whether you're cooking for yourself, your family, or friends, we encourage you to embrace the joy of creating nourishing meals that contribute to your well-being.

As you continue on your path to healthier living, remember to listen to your body, stay connected with your healthcare team, and make choices that support your unique needs and preferences. Small changes can make a big difference, and every step you take towards better health is a step in the right direction.

*Thank you for choosing **"The Psoriatic Arthritis Diet Cookbook"** as your guide. We hope the recipes and insights provided in this book will continue to inspire you to prioritize your health and happiness.*

Wishing you many delicious meals and happy joints on your journey ahead.

Warm regards,

Gustav Henning
Author of "The Psoriatic Arthritis Diet Cookbook: 100+ Recipes for Happy Joints"

www.ingramcontent.com/pod-product-compliance
Lightning Source LLC
Chambersburg PA
CBHW081554250726
48653CB00009B/3432